URGENT
WHISPERS

CARE OF THE DYING

URGENT
WHISPERS

CARE OF THE DYING

*A Personal Reference Manual
for Friends and Family Assisting
A Loved One at the End of Life*

JERRAL SAPIENZA

[signature]

LIFELONG LEARNING
excellence

L L X Press
Eugene, Oregon USA

Published by:

L L X Press

LIFELONG LEARNING EXCELLENCE, INC.

PO Box 380 Eugene, OR 97440-0380 =USA=

in association with
The Bardo of Death Studies
WWW.Bardo.ORG

BOOK DESIGN BY: JERRAL SAPIENZA
COVER ILLUSTRATION: BEVERLY SOASEY
First Edition April, 2002

R93

ISBN: 0-9717107-0-8 Standard Paperback format
ISBN: 0-9717107-5-9 (Spiral) Coil-bound format
Library of Congress Control Number: 2001127217

*For those whose lives have gone before,
they blazed their trails whispering
to those still here behind this door
in urgent hopes we're listening....*

ACKNOWLEDGMENTS

This book has been a labor of love for many years now, and I am deeply indebted to the many friends and family who have patiently stood by me in the process. Notably, thanks to friends Marsha Morrow and Dennis Clark for unflagging support that the book find its way to those who need it, and Portland's Our House AIDS Hospice where Marsha and I first tested some of these ideas. Thanks to editor Holly Saunders for her sensitivity and her reader's eye. Thanks to Elisabeth Kübler-Ross for her pioneering work in death studies. Thanks Patricia Simpson, Stan James, Scott Pengelly, Tasha Beauchamp, Carolyn Janecek and Mary Helen Madrid-Null for early reviews. Beverly Soasey's illustration brought light to the cover. Conari Press' Mary Jane Ryan originally encouraged expansion of exercises which feature prominently in this edition. To my parents John and Fern Sapienza, thanks for persistence that the book find its audience. And thanks to Bob and Maud Corl for their love and knowledge of books. Thanks to my son Adam for just being himself and bringing me great joy. And lastly, the Japanese proverb is thanks to Miho Shimizu of Kobe, Japan.

The book, then, also owes enormous debt to many travelers who in the last twenty years made the first forays to the Other Side with the help of these materials, and in so doing, helped us better understand this incredible awe called death. Thanks to Scott Lucas, co-conspirator in understanding of life through helping out with death. Before his death in 1995 Scott, too, guided many to that Other Shore. And Vern Ho, another tug-boat of the soul, was a mentor whose reflection many of us still miss. Finally, hearty thanks to my grandmother, Jewel Peacock Hegler, for her devotion to the Bible as well as to her nurturing mystical side which afforded support to me in mine. Because of her probing questions about death back in the mid 1980's as she struggled with some of these issues, and her encouragement to trust my intuition and go ahead and write on the subject, this book's seed was planted. As it is harvested now, nearly twenty years later, I have no doubt that she has been helping out from the Other Side since 1991!

Thank You All. -JS   Seattle: Jan 2002

URGENT WHISPERS
CARE OF THE DYING
Table of Contents

URGENT
WHISPERS
CARE OF THE DYING
Introduction

Being present for a friend or loved one in their final days can be an overwhelming and emotionally stressful situation. And yet, these times can also be a special opportunity for us to take stock of our lives, reorder our priorities, and gain some welcome perspective into day-to-day life. Success in the process of attending a friend or loved one at the end of life most often hinges on our ability to pay attention to details, to be able to glean meaning from chaos and disorder, and to just take the time to be truly present, to listen, to care.

Urgent Whispers is a book about caring. It is a book about listening and learning, telling the truth and, something you will hear a lot about in the course of these pages, "just being present in the process." The book also serves as a kind of Quality of Death handbook whose primary role is to offer guidance to friends, family and loved ones in understanding how they can help. It is you, after all, who can best ensure that attention is paid to the interests and communication of your friend or loved one at the end of life.

Audience

Urgent Whispers is for friends and family who will serve as caregivers, and not specifically for the person at the end of life. If your loved one were to choose to read a bit of it early in the process, then it may serve as an ice breaker and conversation starter between the two of you on some of these ideas, but that was not the book's primary intent. Its primary intent was to help you, the caregiver, better understand this process of death and dying.

For tens of thousands of years, death was no stranger to human society. It was merely another common event in the collective fabric of life, dotting every social landscape, touching every family, every age, every class, on a regular basis.

But in these last few decades, especially in the West, most of our societies have tended to push the process of dying away from mainstream life into institutions or hospitals where only a portion of us would come in contact with it at all.

Consequently, as impending death approaches in a family or social structure, the very rarity of it means that many of us simply have no idea what to do, how or where to begin. And the stress of this mystery has certainly had its social cost for family and loved one alike.

Attending death can seem at first glance only a difficult and challenging time. But it can also be so much more than that. For most people, this period can also be an enormously growth-oriented opportunity, even a turning point, harboring some of life's most informative teachers.

If you feel apprehensive and fearful, please realize that you are not alone in these feelings. Most of us have felt very much this way setting foot on this path for the first time. You may be pleasantly surprised later, however, to discover what a learning time this will be and how much you will have learned about yourself and others in the process.

Over the course of this time, try to remain a bit more alert and aware, trusting that everything will make more sense later on. These can be confusing and disorienting times as life patterns and relationships stir, move and change.

As difficult as it may seem right now, try not to worry about yesterday or tomorrow. Instead, try to focus your attention right here, right now, and see if you can be present in this moment. Recognize that the only place you breathe is in the present, not in the past or the future. And if you are able to find peace in this present moment, then breathe it in now.

As you pay attention to the small things in life and their quiet gifts, you may experience a new level of personal reflection from some quite unexpected sources. Try to listen earnestly to these quiet messages, these *urgent whispers*. There are many potential lessons in these times which may help show you a great deal about yourself, about life and living, and about the greater world around you. And do trust that it is not all darkness. There can be magic in these times, too, if we are open to seeing it.

Origins

This collection of *Urgent Whispers* evolved for me over the last twenty years or so, mostly out of my volunteer work with late-stage cancer and AIDS patients, many of whom were courageous, vibrant young people. Before the disease struck they were considered active, intelligent, interesting people, loved by family and friends, living full and involved lives.

But as the disease progressed toward one of the most difficult and challenging times of their lives, a troubling common thread would often emerge. Friends and family often felt confused and overwhelmed, silently fearing they did not know what to do, did not know how to help. And so, in this difficult time when stress and tensions ran high, these same valued friends and family often began to pull quietly away. Disoriented by the process, they often pulled back in confusion and fear, and quite unintentionally nearly abandoned their loved one who lay dying.

That is the tragedy of what happens when we do not trust that we have answers, when our fear of death and fear of doing the wrong thing keeps us from reaching out. That is the main reason I had to write this book. Too many people were not understanding that they already knew what to do.

People have sometimes asked me how I learned these things, what my background is, how I developed my approach at the bedside. Professionally, my initial training was in Education and Engineering, and not in Nursing or Hospice Care. But over the last twenty years I was blessed, or cursed, depending on one's interpretation of the events, with an inordinate number of friends and family who died. Some died of heart attacks or other illnesses, some of suicide, some of accidents. But most died from some degenerative disease like AIDS, cancer, Alzheimer's or ALS.

At first the whole process of death and dying seemed foreign to me, just as it may seem to you. I knew very little about it and I felt unprepared to deal with it. I didn't know what to do or *not* to do. Like so many of us, I wasn't prepared very well earlier in life for dealing with death.

In my early adulthood as death continued to happen around me, I decided I needed to better understand these things. So when I heard about someone else who was nearing death I would take time to go and be with them and see if I could learn to help. Those times were great teachers.

Then another couple of my teachers in this process were two accidents I was involved in, one in January 1984 and the other in August 1987. Both of these resulted in fairly significant trauma to my body. The second one almost killed me. But there was also a gift hidden in each of them, a "near death experience." It is difficult to find words to express just what those experiences meant to me. Certainly they inspired changes. My outlook on life and death and living and dying, for instance, was forever altered. I was gently reminded that difficult times of life are not without their gifts. Since then I have many times been able to reach back into the peace nestled in the trauma of those moments and smile for having lived them.

I encourage you to look back in life and see what messages may have come to you in some of the "Teacher Times" disguised as trauma. Exploring this deep mine of rich resources available to us during our times of yearning, we are often pleasantly surprised by gifts there if we remain receptive. Think back on your life and its challenges. What messages were there? What have you learned? How have you grown?

Getting Started

Being present for a friend or loved one at the end of life is basically just natural human response to a series of natural human events, specifically in this case, the process of death and dying. Were we closer to our social, spiritual and psychological human roots, perhaps even as recently as the past century, we would likely find the work very familiar. There really is no great psychological, spiritual or nursing training necessary to help out in death or to work well with the materials presented in this book.

Mainly what is asked of you is merely to be able to stay focused on the process before you, take note of your options and then make appropriate choices to aid in assisting a friend or loved one's comfort as death approaches.

If you happen to be able to be in attendance at the bedside, then you will find the material here useful as a guide to what your friend is likely to be experiencing. Or if you are reading the material at home or hundreds of miles away from the bedside and not currently directly involved, you may want to use the material as a guide to thinking about what your loved one may be going through and how you might later be of assistance.

Either way, please see **Urgent Whispers** as something of a base camp, a comfortable place to return to when you have a few minutes to yourself and find that you have questions or notations about this process you or your loved one is going through. The book is intended to serve as both reflection and personal accompaniment on your journey. Consider it as a travel planner and guidebook, a companion journal for you with space where you can chronicle what you are feeling and learning, and what you would like to share with others later.

You will find that friends and family may be interested in talking with you about some of your experience, too, to help you both better understand.

Jewel in the Darkness

Make use of the space in the book for your notes, details and observations. During such a flurry of activity as a friend's end of life process you are apt to have a thousand things going through your mind. You may be thinking about contacting people whom you haven't spoken with in years. You may feel like scribbling notes as you talk with someone, recording phone numbers or email addresses of family you need to get in touch with. There is nothing sacred about keeping these pages empty, clean, void of your touch. Notes you put into the book now will be here for you later and will help serve as useful reminders since memory has a way of fading as details pass on by.

Jotting things down as you think of them will be a good way to help review and understand what you have been going through. It will also help give you a head start at dealing appropriately with some of your grief, when you get to that point. The book provides a quiet link back to life through some of the conscious and subconscious ideas you may be processing as you assist in these important times.

In the course of the coming days, you will likely come to a better understanding of death and dying and its natural place in the Bigger Picture, enhancing also an understanding and appreciation for life and living and your place in it all. That is, after all, among the greatest of gifts available to you, and a realistic goal. A renewed appreciation for life and its mystery is one of the most rewarding experiences people often report after being able to spend time with a loved one at the end of life. It is that twinkling jewel in the darkness.

As you are no doubt beginning to realize, the constellation of end of life events and process can sometimes be a dizzying array of confusions. Unfortunately it is sometimes difficult to choose between all the conflicting options and challenges before you. There is no definitive care plan by which you can chart that perfect course home.

Conflicting routines and regimens of vitamins, medicines, therapies, diet; conflicting demands of insurance companies, care providers, legal planners; conflicting pressures of family, friends, neighbors, religious and business associates. These are not simple issues, not easy times. The world can seem off kilter, out of orbit and out of control.

There are many issues which are indeed out of our control and beyond the sphere of our direct influence. As such, we perhaps do best to focus our attention more in places where we *can* make a difference. Certainly one such place is here, just being present for a loved one at the end of life.

We may be called upon to face the reality of the dying process in a variety of challenging ways. Though rewarding, this is not always easy work and it is not always pleasant work. But it is very important work, and we all already know the basics. It is, at its core, merely love and support.

Asking for Help Along the Way

For some people, death and mortality represent mostly fear, panic and hesitation. Superstition, or unrealistic anxiety, sometimes interferes with our ability or desire to understand much about death and dying. It is natural to have apprehensions and anxieties, especially when the source of our stress is that which we tend to label as "the unknown." In such times of stress, it is normal to have shifting feelings of responsibility at any given moment as to what our options are, or how we feel about those options.

Sometimes we may feel like staying close so we do not miss anything and can cherish every precious moment with our loved one. And at other times we may feel almost like running away, trying to get as far away as possible so as to avoid the situation entirely. Confusion and overwhelm can be quite common at complicated times like these.

That said, there is certainly nothing wrong with reaching out and asking for help when you find yourself confused or overwhelmed. The book is designed to help provide you with some kind of guidance you may find useful along the way as well as alternative interpretations for what may be going on around you and what may be expected from you as a friend or caregiver.

But it is very important to be clear that if you are experiencing extreme emotional response to some aspect of what you are going through, it is a good idea to talk to someone. Seek professional help if you need it. A familiar bit of women's wisdom here for some of us (typically men) hesitant to ask for help:

As on life's physical journeys, some folks on these experiential journeys tend to be less willing to ask for directions along the way. But please realize it is okay to ask for help, directions and pointers. You can not always be expected to have maps of everything ingrained in your being, to have all the answers. There is no weakness in asking for help. You are not alone with your questions. Please... Let others help!

Do not hesitate to reach out and find someone to talk to about things. If you do not have an available friend or relative to speak with, grief and counseling resources are often available through local community health services, clinics, or private counselors. Most all people experience some degree of anxiety or stress around death, and it can be exaggerated by other "routine" life stresses. Just being aware of your needs and coping abilities is the best plan. You know best what best works for you in your life.

It is likely you will grow emotionally, spiritually and socially in these times, enriching not only your ability to serve others, but also your ability to better face life's challenges as well. As you experience even small successes they often begin to multiply and your confidence increases your ability to better carry out whatever may be asked of you.

You have embarked here on something of a journey of questioning and understanding. Like a journey in the physical world, you cannot expect to arrive at the same moment you depart. There is still the necessary scenery along the way, its process, timeline and events. It is in the course of that process where you will learn, grow and share with others. Some questions about directions are perfectly normal as you proceed on any journey. It is good and helpful to refer to maps along your way.

As you begin now on this work's journey, reflect again upon what you are undertaking. It is one of the most important roles on the planet, challenging and profound, intensely emotionally stimulating and at its essence, very simply Love. You will surely experience this more and more deeply as you continue.

About the Voice of *Urgent Whispers*

You will notice that in order to avoid the awkward and repetitive usage of he / she or specific personal pronouns, I have adopted here the sometimes unconventional, yet still colloquially common, usage of "they" to refer to the equivalent of she / he.

I also speak sometimes in a collective first-person plural "we" in parts of the book. That is because this book has felt to me, from the very beginning, like a story I was to tell for those who went before. It was their lives and deaths which inspired much of the material here. I believe many of them would have wished this little book could have been available earlier, that their own journey might have been easier. It feels to me now as though we all join together writing this book and offering it to you in love and support.

About the *Whispers* Format

The format of *Urgent Whispers* is dual-paged with an exercise or workspace area on the left page and a brief and often incisive *whisper* at the top of the right, followed by a discussion of how it may be most relevant to you and your loved one. The *whisper* represents a quiet message you may have sensed in the course of your day-to-day vigil assistance, but not quite heard.

With some *whispers* you will notice a greater urgency and they may come across in a somewhat demanding tone. This is intentional. Sometimes there *is* a demanding nature to what may be asked of us. In these times it may be best to pay closer attention to the details of how we help, what we say and how we may be perceived.

Certainly there will be variations on a theme. No one can predict exactly how your friend or loved one may be passing through or responding to some of these stages, concepts or processes. But you will find here many of the useful guideposts along the way.

The *whispers* often represent lessons learned from deaths which may have gone less well, though as their legacy, helped to blaze a trail toward better understanding. The hope is that with these lessons presented as *whispers*, other friends and loved ones will be able to feel more comfortable, more supported, more empowered to die a death on their own terms, peacefully and well cared for. In order to help chart a course, the *whisper* provides you with a small voice of reflection in what otherwise might seem only a difficult space of silence.

As you read a *whisper* or its discussion to yourself or quietly aloud, pause a moment to try to *feel* what its relevant message may be for you in your particular situation: What might your friend or loved one need right now? What might those around you be feeling? What message might you be needing to better understand? What action might be necessary for you to consider?

Vigil Notes and Exercises

For those who like to have a practical exercise to help out, you will find on the left facing page the "Vigil Notes" or "Exercises" where you can more easily interact with the material. By responding to, making notes about, or acting upon the information as presented, it can become more meaningful and applicable to the process.

Consider this left side of the page *your page,* where you can respond to the starter questions or exercises. You can also just write quiet observations, thoughts, memories, to-do notes, or whatever is most useful to you as it comes up. Exercises and sentence-completions are often presented in the first person, starting with an "I" so that you may simply fill in the blank as your own voice, moving as quickly into the idea as possible. Feel free to complete as much or as little as you wish, skipping any which you feel do not apply.

No doubt the vigil process brings up challenging questions. We wonder sometimes where the darkness might lead, or how we will get through it. All of us have asked these questions when we first lost a dear friend, a parent, a spouse, a lover, a family member, a beloved child. We don't yet know where our path leads, yet we know that it stands before us.

See what you can do to participate. The more you are able to interact with the material and respond to situations now, the better overall picture you will have later to return to in the process, when you begin to work through some of the grief and emotion you may wish to express. The exercise pages here are based upon questions and comments others have had at these times which helped them to collect and express important thoughts along the way.

Please consider these materials as something of a torch and compass, gifts perhaps from travelers who have been here before on some of these paths. We offer you these *whispers* now in hopes they might help light your path, lighten your burden, guide you on your way with the kind of reflection *we* ourselves might like to have had available that first time when *we* set out on this path of personal discovery to best tune into our loved one's **Urgent Whispers.**

NOTES:

VIGIL RECORD
In Loving Memory of:

_____

_____

VIGIL NOTES BY

DATES

_____   TO   _____

AT

_____

LOCATION

The essence of what I'm feeling about being here right now is I feel ...

About my friend / loved one, what I feel most right now is ...

The ideal way I would most like to be perceived or represented as I visit here would be ...

Although I may be a variety of things just now, the part of me which I think is most valuable for me to "be here now" is my ...

• *Know that I need you here now. Please just be yourself, taking care that you're taken care of, too.*

Your honest presence is the best and most loving gift you can offer right now. Your friend or loved one deserves that of you. If, as you enter the room, you find yourself trying to pretend to be happy or somehow unaffected by their process, then it is very likely that you are not being yourself. Let your feelings be a cue to you now as to your level of understanding of the process.

A mental state is always contagious to some degree. Honest projection of love and emotion is an important gift. If, at this time, you feel it is difficult for you to be here without feeling overwhelmed with grief and sadness, then perhaps you may want to come back later when you can be more wholly present. Talk to someone. Work things through a bit. Time is of the essence now. You do need to be able to be here, present, as soon as you can.

Do not be too hard on yourself. Feelings of sadness are natural feelings, especially now. All of us are affected by them. Be aware of what the sadness is telling you now:

You and your friend share strong important bonds.

On the short list of things which I'd most like to be able to better understand right now would be...

1)

2)

3)

In order to make myself most useful in being present in the moment, what I can best offer of myself right now to do would be to ...

And what I can consciously try now not to do is...

• Be comfortable while you're with me. Don't make yourself uncomfortable doing what you cannot do.

It is common to feel uncomfortable about your usefulness in times like these. If you find yourself pretending to be comfortable, then you probably are not. If you are capable of helping out with the personal care of your loved one, then feel free to be as helpful as you can, without interfering with any professional care also in attendance. If you feel unable to be of direct assistance, then it is probably best that you do not try to do so. You could actually make things more difficult and contribute to discomfort in the process. Knowing when to ask for help is, in itself, something useful, too.

This is not meant, however, to discourage you from finding a way to help. Basic care can be attended by anyone. You can straighten the blankets, fluff the pillows, make sure there is fresh water or facial tissue near. But be mindful of making a commotion in the process. Move slowly and peacefully. Speak soothingly as you communicate with your loved one. Keeping their room cleaned up and tidy can help maintain the feeling of control and comfort. Advice my grandmother used to offer at times like these:

"Make yourself useful as well as ornamental."

You can perhaps feel more comfortable, just doing what feels natural as you make yourself useful now.

Do I understand the concept of "Breath Budget?"

(Bear in mind that some people don't like to be asked a lot of questions... pay attention to how you are received. Be especially aware of whether or not your questions seem to be pestering.)

Questions I have asked and responses I received:

Questions I would like to remember to ask later:

• *Feel free to ask me what I want, what I feel, what I need. Then honor and respect my answer, or my silence.*

It is important that you check in with your loved one to get a better idea of their needs, wants, desires. When genuine, your checking in can help them feel more in control, more loved and appreciated. Ask. You may want to word things in a format more akin to Yes/No, especially if your loved one is not speaking very much any more.

Be helpful, without pestering. It is important not to ask something merely for the sake of asking. Sometimes silence has its place, too. Be patient if your questions are met with silence. Let silence pass comfortably.

You may have an answer much later. If not, silence itself may be an answer as well. It may mean that you need to take a break from asking questions, or that on a Breath Budget, complicated questions are just too difficult to answer now. Speak softly, but clearly, and try to be sensitive. Perhaps you can *feel* some of the answers. Take your cue from them.

Be patient. Listen with your heart. Hold a hand.

If today were *my* last day to live, what issues might I need yet to resolve?

What incompletions must I yet complete?

What skill have I not yet learned or taken up which I always wanted to?

What travel have I yet to do?   Where shall I go?

What important messages must I still deliver soon?

Where shall I begin?!

• *Priorities look so very different from the end of life. I wish I had realized this before.*

These are times of reflection. As life comes to a close, people usually look back and review memories, often considering alternatives to what they did or did not do during the course of their lives.

Usually it is not their possessions which matter now. Not how big the house, not how fast the car, not whether things were always neat and clean. No concerns any more of that best parking space at work.

All those extra hours worked, whether we dressed in the latest fashion, whether we kept up with the Jones'... None of these matter any more from the larger over-view of True Priorities. The kinds of things which do seem to concern folks more at the end of life:

I wish I had learned to dance / fly / play the piano.
I wish I had been more kind to ___.
I wish I had taken that trip to ___.
Why didn't I spend more time with ___?
Does ___ know I love him / her?
Will my family be taken care of?

Regrets are teachers too. A regret is a concern which was too busy, too fearful, or too proud to *just be*.

Any changes you'd like to make about now?

Is there anyone here (myself included) who may be performing the duties of "gatekeeper" just now?

How do I feel about these duties, or this person?

Exercise for the Gatekeeper:
An important consideration of a gate is to keep something in or keep something out. Which is it here?

Might I have control issues around being gatekeeper?

Is there anyone who might rightfully or wrongfully perceive me now to be meddling in their affairs?

Am I responsibly protecting my loved one right now from potentially difficult people or situations? How?

Who can independently help me to see if I'm being a fair and appropriately responsible gatekeeper?

• *I may have need of a gatekeeper now, but I also need to have time with my family and friends.*

Ideally, the gatekeeper issue should be considered early in the process, and may be a "team" rather than just one person. Best to take a cue from the loved one on this issue. Those who were always rather gregarious with lots of friends around may tend to want to be more private when confined to a bed. Or they may want to still have as many visitors as possible. Check in with them often and find out.

Symbolic Duties of the Gatekeeper may include...
Sergeant at Arms: Help monitor traffic and ensure that people don't overstay their welcome. Some people may not be welcome at all just now for a variety of reasons. Keep an eye out to see which.

Appointment secretary: Help look up and invite in any chosen friends or family whom they have not yet been able to visit with but may still like to see.

Overseer / Manager: It's probably a good idea to pop in periodically even in "closed meetings," to ensure personal care needs are being met and all is well.

Gatekeepers should be sensitive and responsible in directing traffic, yet try not to meddle either.

It's a tightrope act to be a good gatekeeper
and sometimes just about as dangerous!

How do I truly feel about the diagnosis, the process, this end of life care before me?

Is the diagnosis clear to my friend or loved one?

Am I able to understand and accept the diagnosis?

Are there ways in which I may tend not to want to be honest, either in my words or in my actions?

If I had questions, who might help me understand?

• You probably don't need to protect me from the truth.

Death can be a strange time when people sometimes feel that they need to protect the dying party from the truth. Stereotypically, this is envisioned as a doctor who speaks candidly with relatives about a patient's condition, yet not with the patient directly.

In some cultures it can be quite common for the doctor not to speak so directly of these things. If that is the case, then it may be left more to family and friends to make the decision how much or when to talk about the diagnosis.

If you find yourself in a quandary as to what to say and what not to say when you speak with your loved one, perhaps the best plan is merely to commit to be open to discussing things at any time your loved one may ask, at any point in the process. Take your cues from them.

It is very rare when a dying loved one is not aware of their condition. They may not speak directly about it for any number of reasons, but they probably do know.

If you hone your listening skills to pay close attention to your loved one's words and style of communication, you will know what to discuss, and what not to.

Sometimes the truth takes all day to tell.
Sometimes it is a single word.

What do I know about this disease and how it affects the body?   What else might I need to know about symptoms or progression of the disease?

Do I need to seek more outside help with personal care needs or general procedures?
If so, then where might I find answers?

I remember before the illness, a whole, happy, healthy, active being. A couple of my fondest memories I have of us together which can help me to keep alive a better perspective :

1)

2)

• *Treat my body with dignity. It is part, not all, of me.*

End of life progressions can significantly change a person. Degenerative diseases continue to weaken the body and a dying person can feel significant loss of self-respect, autonomy and dignity. There can also be tremendous pain, feelings of helplessness, and not wanting to be a burden to family or social system during this process of the body weakening, faltering and failing.

How you relate to your loved one now and how you show your compassionate support is very important. Ideally, they need to recognize your love and respect. They need to feel sincerity in your presence, and know that you do understand that they *not* just an illness and are so much more than *just* the body.

Personal hygienic care at the end of life is disturbing to some caregivers. If it disturbs you, then perhaps it is best that you know how to ask for help and when to leave certain procedures to others who can better be in attendance of your loved one's hygienic needs. Either way, it is important that those present conduct themselves with attention to the highest respect and dignity for the body and the being. This whole and wonderful loving being has a *body* which is ill.

See with your memory,
See with your heart.
Open to love.

No doubt I will soon enough have an opportunity to move deeper into and through Grief and back to life in the process. But for now:

What I can best do to be of help in the transition is . . .

For later: Notes about my thoughts of Denial / Anger / Resentment / Bargaining with Death / Acceptance *(Elisabeth Kübler-Ross's classic stages of grief.)*

• *Please do not grieve for me now. Grieving is for yourselves later.*

When you come to be in attendance with someone in the end-of-life process, this is not the time to grieve. There will be plenty of time later for grieving. This is not the most productive use of your time and energy just now.

Sometimes people will visit a dying person and un-thinkingly choose to behave as though they feel a need to try to demonstrate some great sadness and grief. Perhaps they believe that they are showing their love and respect by how affected they will be after their loved one is gone. But there are many better ways to spend this time, to share these precious moments.

Recall that your loved one is still here and needs you in the present, right here, right now. Grieving is typically past-centered. You can best attend to your grieving at a later point in the process when your loved one no longer has physical and emotional needs of you.

There is still a part of that difficult trail yet to go, and that is what you are here to aid in supporting.

Bring yourself to the present now.
Hold a hand.
Smile.

Do I know the difference between feelings of *pity* and feelings of *compassion*?

When did I last feel *pity or pitied*?

What did it feel like?

When did I last feel *compassion* for or from another?

What did that feel like?

When reading the paragraph across the page, was my breathing deep and full or shallow and tight?

How can I best ensure that I truly bring and project only *compassion*?

• Do not bring me your pity. Bring me your honest compassion and expression of love, or bring me nothing.

Your state of mind is extremely important while you are visiting with your friend. There is a significant and noticeable difference between feelings of pity and feelings of compassion which may accompany you.

Compassion is a grand gift of open commitment and awareness you agree to live in, an emotional state of acceptance and willingness to try and understand, to be of service, to learn and grow from the experience.

Pity, on the other hand, is so very different. It is a close-in contagion of fear which requires that you shrink in order to fit into it, focusing all of your attention first on your worries of someone else's situation, then on how you project this onto your own superstitions of Life and Death. It fears prolonging the experience.

Be conscious of your breathing right now as you are reading this paragraph. Is it deep and full and open? Or is it shallow and tight and cautious? If you can be more aware of your breathing and try to keep it open and full and hearty, you will find the gentle space of compassion more easily, more often.

Compassion opens to possibility and breathes deeply.
Pity closes in with fear and breathes shallowly.
Seek to be more open, aware and joyful.

Looking back at our relationship, some of the ways in which I might still be harboring feelings of resentment, abandonment or fear of loss of control would be:

Are there issues I might still need to emotionally work through in order to be more present?

How might I have a tendency to try to *take* right now, and how might I ensure that I do *not* do so?

• *Do not come here to take from me. I need my energy now more than ever.*

It may seem obvious to suggest that now is not the time to be "taking." But with emotions running so high during the end of life process, unconscious feelings of resentment, abandonment or loss of control on the part of family and visitors can result in behaviors which can be very draining for your friend or loved one just now.

This is not the best time or place to come to the bedside and try to make a final peace or kneel and cry, or apologize or beg forgiveness. Neither is it the time or place to seek any particular indication of absolution or acceptance. Earlier in the process, when the person is cogent, responsive and stronger, these things can be achieved, or can be at least brought up. But not now.

As the end of life process continues, a loved one will slip further and further away, absorbed in their own process of resolution and preparedness, with very little energy available for much else. This is not the place for seeking to receive any message or for reliving or relieving past difficulties, grudges, misunderstandings.

Try best to be a supportive vessel of
Love, Peace and Understanding.

Am I still in denial about death?   How can I know?

Am I ready for this?   What makes me think so / not?

How might I better deal with the truth now and help in the process of resolution?

• *Do not be afraid to admit that I am dying.*

Being able to admit to yourself that your friend or loved one is dying is a first step toward understanding the realities of the death process. To the dying person, the dying process is clearly never very far away from their awareness, even if certain aspects of the details may still seem to be rather mysterious.

This does not mean that you necessarily need to talk to your friend or loved one here about dying or about the process. Simply take your cue from them.

Once a terminal disease advances beyond a certain stage, there is little point in trying to avoid the fact that death is imminent. It may seem difficult to admit the possibility of finality "so soon." This is likely due to fear or habit, unable to imagine a world with your friend or loved one no longer present.

The important thing now is that the more time you lose dealing with the truth, the more time is stolen from the precious necessity of resolution. And this stage of resolution and completion is very important.

As you are able to consciously be here now with an open and understanding mind, so you are a valuable part of your friend's process.

> Don't hurry understanding or discussion
> but don't delay it either.

Am I indeed able to say that I feel I am okay and taken care of?

Not that I necessarily need to say anything aloud, but given the situation, how *will* I manage and how *will* these responsibilities be taken care of?

1)

2)

3)

In what ways might I be trying to hold on right now, not having given assurances that we will be okay?

• *I need to know that you will be okay as I leave you. How will you manage? Are you taken care of?*

There are many things on your loved one's mind in this process of closing down, resolving and putting things in order.

Think what it must be like, to know that your life is coming to a close now, that the important things you have taken care of all these years, all your dreams, your works, your family, your friends... all must be left here.

There is often a difficulty in letting go of the responsible feelings which have gone along with their role here. You can make things easier right now by assuring your loved one that these responsibilities will be tended.

Remember that it is important not to trivialize perceived importance of their concerns, even if you feel they may be placing undue importance on things you can easily handle. It is not you right now who needs this peace.

You can help in the process of easing these troubling burdens, by reminding your loved one that you will be okay as you are left here, that you have _____ to look after you, that, though you appreciate their loving devotion, it is not necessary now that they delay their needs, worrying about you.

Your reassurance helps.

Am I aware of any changes in food preferences now or changes which we might wish to consider making?

When we talk about food desires and needs, what I am learning is:

What seems to be working, or what is not working?

From what I've learned, are there foods I need to see if I can find?

Are there foods which I need to make sure are *not* brought in due to preference, reaction or request?

• Do not try to feed me what I choose not to eat, nor keep me from eating what I want. My dying body has different needs and desires than my living body.

As caregivers, friends and family of a dying person, it is important to realize that sometimes you may find yourself in the unenviable and uncomfortable position of trying to find *something* which will have a little appetite responsiveness and will draw out a pleasant reaction from your loved one. Sometimes even the smell of food or cooking anywhere near is repulsive. You may even have to keep a fan running to keep "unpleasant" odors from entering this area.

Or, on the other hand, you may find yourself being asked for cravings you never even knew they liked. Either way, don't try to interpret or challenge their desires. Take your best cues now from the present, and not the past, as to what is most appetizing. There is no reason to impose any new kind of dietary restrictions except what is absolutely necessary. The more control of diet they can maintain, the better.

Sour fruit, cough drops, ice chips, cucumber, fruit or fruit juice may be special favorites now since they help "quietly" keep the mouth moist and clean tasting. Helping keep the teeth and mouth clean and the lips moist will also go a long way toward comfort.

An occasional meal of your own at the bedside can help maintain a family feeling at mealtimes, too.

When I look around the room with more than just my eyes, I can try to be aware of the subtle senses, too. Some of what I notice here is:

Verbal or non-verbal cues that something may be bothersome here and may need to be changed:

How's the room temperature and air flow?
Too warm?   Too cool?   Too stuffy?

• *Be aware that I may be more sensitive to Light, Sound, Smell and Touch. I am dying, but I am not yet gone.*

As death approaches, the sense of hearing is often the last to be impaired, although there may also be a heightening of some of the other senses as well. Be especially considerate if you should rub on lotions or massage your loved one. Be mindful of adjustments in temperature, lighting and sound. Best said:

Just be sensitive and take nothing for granted.

Perhaps the most obvious way you might notice a sensitivity to sound is when your loved one startles, jumps or cringes when you move suddenly or make loud sounds.

Maintain a special sensitivity to noises such as rattling utensils, medical apparatus, bedside gadgetry, etc. when you are helping out around the room.

It is most disconcerting for people to learn the hard way that their loved one was not exactly sleeping or unconscious all the while. Contrary to what you and other visitors may think, conversations may very well not only be overheard, but comprehended and reported back to you later.

Be sensitive and respectful at all times.

Have we discussed flowers?   Perhaps favorites?

If so, what I have learned about likes / dislikes and the nature of these flowers' tendency to be beautiful without overpowering...

Checking around the room and bedside regarding any particularly overpowering smells from flowers or anything else, what I find is:

Any visitors I know of whom I have noticed come in a little strongly perfumed?

How is *my* personal "bouquet" or "perfume level?"

• Be aware that flowers and perfumes can be over-powering and that my senses may be offended.

Persons in late-stage degenerative diseases will often have some degree of difficulty breathing and can be significantly affected by strong perfumes or fragrant flowers introduced into their environment.

Well-meaning visitors who bring in beautiful fragrant flowers, or who dab on a bit too much perfume before coming to visit, may be far less welcome than had they come less adorned.

It is important to be aware that strong fragrances (as well as odors of cigarette smoke, candles or incense) can be overwhelming even to the strong and healthy. Certainly the situation can be greatly exaggerated when the body is weakened and can be particularly unpleasant.

If you are in any doubt, you may wish to check some-one else's impressions before getting too close. And be aware from the perspective of *the person in bed.*

Flowers can certainly be pleasant and beautiful gifts for those who have an appreciation for them. But some flowers' potentially strong fragrances can also be quite distractive right now. Try to be aware of extremes.

Beauty never overpowers.

If someone were to be watching me from across the room or down the hall, how would I appear?

What could someone perhaps tell about me?

How are my interpersonal skills / bedside manner?

• *Come sit down here with me instead of so far away.
I can see and hear you better if you are at my level.*

Though hearing is usually the last of the senses to go,
sight can be one of the first impaired. Coming closer
allows you to be sure you connect. It's often possible
to tell how comfortable a caregiver is from clear across
the room or down the hall, simply by seeing how close
they're willing to be to the bed and what the body
language looks like while they're at the bedside. Try
to be open, honest and compassionate.

Remember that it is very unlikely that your friend will
infect you or in any way put you at risk by your coming
closer. Yet it can make a world of difference to them
if you will be nearer, for practical reasons as well as
personal ones.

From a practical perspective, the nearer you are the
less energy has to go into communicating with or
understanding you. When you are near enough you
are best seen, heard, touched and understood.

From a personal perspective, a special bond between
you deserves closer proximity. If indeed the two of
you are close friends or family members, then it is easy
to see why your being nearer can help them to feel
more special, loved and taken care of.

> Share with your friend as an equal,
> a reminder of how you care.

In order that I keep my life intact and still be able to comfortably and supportively be here, what "shifts" am I able to commit to keeping?

Where else might I be able to seek help with shifts?

Who might wish to help out, or who would be able?

Who else already commits to other "vigil watch-times?"

What are my current feelings around self-judgment, expectation, guilt and resentment about being here or not being able to be here?

• *Stay with me only if you can do so freely.*

One thing which is often helpful to a loved one in late-stage degenerative disease is for there to be a familiar face, familiar voice, familiar touch always near, all around the clock. That often means that family or friends will organize a vigil and different people or teams will take different watch-times on the vigil.

Be mindful of agreeing to take a watch you cannot follow through on. If, for instance, you try to stay for an extended period such as an overnight visit yet really do not have the energy it may take to do so, this is apt to foster resentment on both ends. You may begin to resent a draining of energy that you do not have, and your friend will begin to resent your lack of presence since, though you are here, you are mostly just taking up physical and emotional space.

This is a crucial time of your friend's need for resolution and nurturance. For this, a space of safety and comfort, love and support is necessary. Feel free to help if you can, by offering to tend some of that time.

If your being there too long is a concern, perhaps shorter visits are more appropriate so that you might be able to be more wholly present, now and later.

The gift of sitting vigil
can be a gift of peace to you both.

How might I better be supportive right now, instead of just having a long, sad face?

What wonderful memories can I call upon inside just now, to help me think about a moment when we shared some particularly fine times?

Where were we when we last shared a beautiful time or a warm moment of true friendship's bond? I can be there in my mind again and perhaps bring back that moment ...

• *Why do you look at me so sadly? Yes, I may be in pain, but your focusing on it doesn't help.*

Though you may feel you want to be aware of what your friend is undergoing, you may not be aware of your friend's awareness of *you*. Certainly there is less communication as the process of death deepens. How you present yourself now is important. Try to get beyond heavy, dark and difficult sadness. Yes, this is a difficult time. But relief is coming, and that is good.

It would be wonderful for you to try to be present in an honest feeling of lightness and love if you can. Consider a feeling of compassion, wherein you might be as a candle in their darkness.

Offer your love and light that your friend might know less darkness. Imagine being lost in a dark and dismal pain, or a blurry confusion and helplessness. What better gift from someone at a time like that than the gift of a light and loving heart?

Not that you should pretend. Far from it. Merely reach into your memories and find some wonderful moment you have shared with them, a gentle laugh, a beautiful day, a childhood joy, moments of peace. Recall those.

A quiet shared memory can be a
welcome twinkling light in the darkness.

Which caregiver traits seem most helpful now, and how do they make a difference?

Are there things I might learn from the gentle and comforting ways of other caregivers whom I've seen?

Are there certain distractive processes or movements I need to be more aware of?

Am I conscious of any commotion I might cause?

• *Please inform me what you're doing to my body so I better understand the process.*

This is true for all kinds of caregiving. Whenever you are taking care of someone in any stage of any disease or disability, it is a good idea to make a practice of always informing them what it is you're doing or about to do to their body, so as to help alleviate the stress and anxiety associated with the process.

"I'm just going to tuck you in a bit now and adjust your pillow. There. Is that okay?"

Please consider what it feels like. It is not always easy to be dependent, to have someone else taking care of you. It may be difficult sometimes to understand who is doing what, when, how and why.

As a healthy able-bodied person they very likely would have realized everything going on. But complications of the disease and side-effects of medications can cause the mind to blur and understanding to slow.

Consider how you might like to be treated.
Be gentle. Be patient. Be kind.

Regarding the general relaxation qualities of this place, does this room seem to be the kind of environment in which I could relax?

What seems to help? What seems to distract?

Regarding music, nature sounds, waterfall or other ambience for the space here, what has seemed to work, and what has not seemed to work so far:

(You should be careful assuming you know what music they want to hear. As with food, just because history suggested they liked music "X" before, that pattern may not still apply. Recall that a dying body has very different needs, desires and tolerances than a living body. Quiet relaxation music is usually best.)

• *Everything seems so distracting to me now. Can you help me to relax?*

The hectic nature of personal care, and the constant flow of visitors (or lack of them) can make it very difficult for persons in late-stage to get much of a feeling of relaxation and peace, whether they are at home, in hospice care or in a hospital.

It might be a good idea to have quiet music or a small trickling waterfall in the room to help relieve some of the nervous stress. Such sounds can be very peaceful, provided the music is appropriate and the waterfall does not run low on water. Take note of your loved one's reactions and make sure the music and / or waterfall sounds are appreciated as truly relaxing and pleasant.

"Relaxation" or "Ambient" music will usually be the best choice in music, even when your loved one tended to listen to very different kinds than these. When playing music, play it very softly so it is barely audible at all. It serves the purpose of calming the subconscious and providing a current of love and musical spirit on which to lean for a little more support. Its peaceful current can be like a gentle stream flowing through the room, helping your loved one to relax.

> This quiet current of sound can also be
> soothing for visitors and caregivers.

Am I certain I know what their preferred spiritual values / religious doctrines are?

Have we spoken about it specifically?

Who is their spiritual leader / primary contact?

How might I contact that person or organization?

Is there someone else whom I might contact who shares these particular religious beliefs or spiritual values?

• *Please respect my own religious beliefs, whether they are consistent with yours or not.*

There is sometimes a temptation by some people to believe that they know best how to proceed with the rites and ceremonies surrounding the death process of a loved one, whether this is consistent with the loved one's belief system or not.

But it is *inexcusable* to ignore the wishes of your friend or loved one. It is important that you do not pressure them or their process to conform to your beliefs or expectations in these final days, any more than you would like to be so pressured on your death-bed by someone of another belief system.

Not that you should be required to approve of, or even understand, their particular religious or spiritual beliefs (or lack of them). But it is imperative that regardless of your beliefs, the process now must depend on the wishes and beliefs of your friend or loved one, not yours.

If by chance you were fortunate enough to share their particular religion, denomination or beliefs, then so much the better. You may be of particular value in their assistance now. Either way, it is good to be aware of differences in belief systems around you.

Sometimes your beliefs will draw others closer.
Sometimes they will push others away.
Are you aware of which is the case now?

What are the primary religious / spiritual beliefs of my friend or loved one here?

How do my specific religious / spiritual beliefs differ from my friend or loved one's around end-of-life rites, practices, prayer, or devotions?

What might I still need to know in order to be sensitive to their particular beliefs regarding visions of the Other Side, Deities, Judgment, Forgiveness or other rituals?

Is there room in my own beliefs to be able to accept beliefs significantly different from my own?

• *Please do not demean nor mock nor cry out against my own views and practices of Spirit. They are mine.*

It is important not to make assumptions about belief systems. How you were raised could differ from what you believe now. What you believe now could differ from what someone else believes now as well as how they were raised. Belief systems are very personal.

Unless you are certain that your belief systems match, it is probably best that you keep beliefs, chants, prayers, invocations and ceremonies to yourself as much as possible. Even though you may only want to help, what you do must be appropriate spiritual help *from their perspective* or you may do more harm than good! Not all spiritual beliefs are identical or applicable, and you must take your cues from the bed in order to be most useful in the process.

Perhaps it is best to consider that not all beliefs, visions, expectations and practices are universal. It is important that you be willing to be open to another possibility of how spirit works in someone else's life and honor their desires and choices.

Spiritual beliefs can vary greatly.
Open to faith and wisdom.

Regarding the web of Friendship, Family and Folks I've connected with here, some stories I have heard include:

(Date / Who / Narrative of the Story ...)

• *Learn about some of the parts of my life you may not have known anything about.*

In order that you better understand your loved one, it is a good idea for you to visit with some of the other people who have also come forward at this time.

Interactive and social traffic in the same room here may be distractive. Always remember your first duty is to support and comfort care, and not to socializing.

It is a comforting gesture for you to be interested in the life of your friend. Surely there are aspects of that story which you know little about which may be filled in a bit by speaking with some of the other family, friends and associates who may come forth now.

You are likely to find that they, too, appreciate the sharing of the story. The companionship of being able to talk to someone else who feels similarly about your special friend may bring the two of you together and help you both learn and grow.

Share the bounty of friendship's gifts.

There have been many private shared moments and wonderful memories which are special to us both. As I reflect back now, three of the memories I am most happy we have been able to share include:

1)

2)

3)

The kinds of things which seemed to best help us to be happy while we were together were:

How might we share some part of that again now?

Of the children I have seen here _____, what they seem to be thinking of it all, and how are they dealing with the situation seems to be:

• *Be as pleasant and present as possible while you're with me. Be happy that you are here for me.*

It is perhaps difficult to recognize opportunity for being happy, pleasant and patient now as you accompany your friend or loved one to death's door. And it is perfectly natural for you to feel frustrated, confused, helpless and fearful about doing the right thing now.

But try to relax a bit. Try to be yourself. Be at peace as much as possible and remember that your gentle, patient presence is exactly the kind of love and support which can be most meaningful for your loved one now.

There is a comfortable presence in merely sharing time with someone who needs you and whom you help so easily and so well. This is a subtle kind of happiness you both need right now, bountiful and pure, which pours over you merely as a gift in the moment.

Children are especially good at being able to live in this kind of happiness, since they haven't yet learned *not* to be happy. Especially if children were always a big part of life, it is important for them to be able to continue to share now. Try not to unnecessarily shield children from sharing these special times. But do help them to mindfully be more calm and respectful.

> Trust that this moment can offer you cues
> as to how happiness is best expressed.

Are there issues I still need to clear in order for us to be completely at peace?

Are there other family members or friends here who might help me to clear some of my issues? Perhaps I can also help some of them clear some of theirs?

Exercise:
Try writing a GoodBye Letter as though you were really going to give it to them or speak those words. (Just keep this one to yourself.) But what might you need to include in that letter if you were *really* going to be sending it?

• *Clear your grudges before you come to clear with me. Do your goodbyes twice if necessary, once alone and once with me.*

Remember that your loved one needs as much support and strength as possible for this end of life process. It is important that if you have a grudge or issue with them, now is *not* likely the time to expect to be doing anything about it.

This is a good time to come and say goodbye. But make sure that there is no undercurrent of needing also to clear long-held, deeply-felt emotional issues, attachments or grudges. This is not the time.

If you strongly feel it necessary to clear certain issues, then do so on your own time at home in your own space, by writing an unsent letter, or ranting and raving at a pillow, or whatever similar means you have to release your emotion in a place which is safe for you and your loved ones. This is a much kinder, yet still effective, way to express your emotions and vent your anger, rage and resentment without having to vent on your friends or loved ones.

Ironically, this private and personal way of processing emotions can sometimes give you an eerie feeling that the message gets across anyway. It does work.

If I am having trouble relaxing and being present, what makes it difficult for me to be able to "just be" right now?

What would help me (or others) to better tune in, or stay more present?

Exercise:
Vigil Sitting is an age-old practice of person-to-person ritual. Imagine your friend, yourself, the bed, all in a room somewhere in an age-old society, five hundred or even five thousand years ago. There are no modern devices, no magazines, no news reports, no games. Just the two of you together in a quiet time of peace.

In such a situation, what might you have said or done as evidence of the importance of your relationship? Could you not, then, as easily communicate the same message the same way here and now?

• Don't come to visit me only to read, sew, watch TV, chat with each other or write letters. I need your loving presence, attention and commitment here as I let go. Or I may prefer to have my space.

This can be difficult for some people, especially well-meaning but fearful parents, siblings or children who mask their discomfort "doing" things in order to try and forget the non-routine of the situation. But recall that your loved one is in a very non-routine situation right now, too. Do not take that lightly.

Be aware that, especially in late-stage, a loved one's room is not a good place for you to nervously "do." It can be too distracting for them since they often need to conserve energy and let go. If earlier on, *they* want you to read to them, or watch tv with them, or play cards, take your cue from them. Remember that you will, on your own, have plenty of time later for "doing." Here, now, "being" is most important. Try to pay attention to subtle communication and needs.

How to avoid the "do" tendency? Stay close. Hold a hand. Stroke back the hair. Smile. Sing quietly. Kiss your friend lightly on the cheek, if that was your relationship. Put lotion on their arms or legs. Help keep their lips moist with water, if they want it.

Be present, yet be willing to give some space
if things get too irritable with activity.
See and Feel with your Heart.

If I were the one in this bed right now, what might I be feeling about now?

What things do I know would be important to me?

What might I like my visitors to be aware of?

What changes might I want to make?

Exercise:
While your friend sleeps a bit or is resting quietly, watch the rise and fall of their chest. Tune into that rhythm of their breath. Match your breathing with theirs and pay attention to what you then feel.

What I feel is:

• *Tune into what I'm going through here. Be present with me here and now.*

It is not an unreasonable request that you should, as much as possible, attempt to be present in the here and now and tune into what is happening with your loved one while you are physically in their presence.

Dying is a very difficult process in some ways and extraordinarily simple in others. Not all folks let go as easily. During late stage, the process of dying is, in many ways, just agreeing to let go.

If you were close to your loved one and recall how they dealt with control issues earlier in life, then you likely also have a pretty good idea how they may deal with letting go now. Letting go in life is usually similar to letting go in death, in that it is merely a process of disengaging from the struggle.

If you can "tune in" and be present with your friend without trying to pull them back to be with you, this is some of the best support you can offer just now.

Especially during these later stages, try being still and listening carefully, breathing with them in unison. This can be a very effective method of getting in touch, feeling more of what is happening with them.

Love unconditionally.
Remember wonderful times.

Stories of this Essential Friend / Loved One I know:

Exercise:
If I were to organize a Memorial Celebration and wanted to share certain representative memories, some of the stories I could tell might include:
[Humor? / Childhood? / Travels? / Accolades?]

1)

2)

3)

4)

• Please commit to remember me. Share me. Become my essence for someone who did not know me.

It is comforting for your loved one to know that they will not be forgotten. It is nice to know one's work, ideas, loves, aspirations, sense of humor, beliefs and gifts live on beyond this life.

One way of sharing and becoming their essence is by telling their story, verbally or in writing. Begin it now, if you wish. Tell it in as significant a way as possible, with as much detail and connectedness as you can.

This is the essential function of eulogies after death, obituaries, headstones, epitaphs, memorials, wakes, funerals, trees planted, poems written, gatherings and celebrations. All these share gifts with the living, too.

For those at the end of life, it is very important to be able to know that someone remembers, that life was not in vain, that life's work yet continues. It is a great comfort and relief to know that there are still those here on this side of the veil who will be able to carry on the passion, the meaning, the sharing of this ebbing life's story.

Commit to remember. Commit to love.
Commit to share.

Regarding people I have met in the process, what has been their most interesting aspect to me?

What has been the most challenging aspect of trying to just be here and be non-judgmental right now?

Do I find myself judging certain people or personalities here now? If so, do I know why?

Are there specific people, groups, or behaviors around which I am finding myself most uncomfortable? Why might that be the case?

Is it possible that I might also be irritating others or pushing their buttons? How?

• *Please honor my love for my friends and my family, even if you don't know them, understand them or feel close to them yourself.*

There is, as we can readily see, an unending variety of personalities on the planet. It is almost certain that you do not know all of your friends' friends. It should come as no surprise, then, that you may also find yourself meeting some new people here, in the course of being available for your dying loved one now.

It is also possible that you may not like, or may not understand, some of the people you will meet. And that is okay. But please try to remember that these are times for acceptance and resolution. Just because these people are someone else's family or friends, they do not necessarily have to be yours.

General respect works well for this situation. Recall that you may never see some of these people again and they likely feel as strongly for your friend as you do. Perhaps it is best for all to just try and get along and be pleasant as much as possible. Emotions and judgments can strain at times like these.

Be good to yourself and to others:

Take care and breathe deeply,
trying to keep an open mind.

(These things may not come quite clear just yet. You may wish to re-visit this question in a few days, weeks or months to review some of the "strange coincidences" with people you met, what you learned about each other, etc.)

Notes on coincidences / synchronicities surrounding any of the people I have met here or events as they have unfolded:

What new friendships have I noticed evolving here?

• *Open to new people who may come to be present in my death. Share with one another.*

Often there can seem a sense of synchronicity in the appearance of people and events surrounding someone's impending death. People may appear whom you may have known little or nothing about, yet who feel almost completely familiar. And others whom you know, but have not seen in years, may feel to you as though you just saw them yesterday. The fabric of time seems to knit together differently in times like this.

It is not uncommon to forge strong new bonds of friendship in the course of attending the death of a significant friend, family member or lover. This time offers many opportunities for people from different origins to come together, as a single new community of purpose, and learn and grow in the process.

Perhaps not surprisingly, this synchronicity and blend of lives is often seen as the work of the loved one, silently and passively bringing new friends together. As you meet people and get to know one another during the course of your common vigil, you may find that new ties emerge from these alliances which also happen to carry on some of your friend's life's work.

Maybe there are no accidents,
And all things were meant to be?

What deeper issues am I better understanding from being able to be here in my loved one's death process?

What parts of our relationship am I letting go of now, in the process of this death?

In what ways am I aware of the unity of this friendship bond? How were we as One?

What part of that unity remains here with me still?

• Take the time to reflect on what part of yourself dies with me. How does our relationship benefit us both?

Realize that each of us has something to learn from death as friends and family members die around us. We, just as they, learn something about letting go and redefining relationship. We also begin to realize that each of us is part of the ongoing flow of humanity and that our time, too, will come.

It is not easy to prepare to leave now and give up all of these friendships and relationships they have known all their life. One comforting thought for the dying person is to know that a part of what the two of you shared will accompany them on their journey, just as a part of what you shared will remain here with you.

There is often an uneasiness about death and the prospect of having to go it alone. Ultimately each of us is born alone and will die alone. Yet the precious moments and comforts of life and living are usually in the presence of our friends and family.

Life is significantly enriched by love, affection, touch and companionship. These are gifts we give one another in support along the way. Friends, family and memories are all important.

Be this for your friend now:
Quiet, Connected, Available.

The support situations and people which are helping me right now to survive and to cope are:

Some of the dormant issues or creative insights which have come up for me in this time include:

• *Talk or write about your feelings when you go home.*

Your feelings right now are important and it is a good idea for you to have some kind of a useful support system which encourages your working through and processing some of the feelings which may come up.

Take note of all your feelings, but pay special attention to those around resentment, abandonment, pain, fear, expectations and issues of love and companionship.

Feelings and memories can be stirred up in these times which you have not felt or thought about in years. It will probably help if you can open to these ideas as they emerge. Try to process them in some way. You may want to talk with a close friend or confidant or write a bit in a journal about your feelings. This will help you recharge between visits so that when you return here you can be more emotionally as well as physically present for your friend or loved one.

Whatever support method you have available, try to continue to express yourself throughout the process. Feel free to begin it here, on the left side of the page. Later when you look back and visit these writings and notes you will appreciate their gifts.

Let your reflections be little time capsules,
timely peace offerings of the process
which you gave yourself for later.

Exercise: Try a clear, gentle greeting as you arrive:

"Good Morning, Emily.   It's Steve here.

...pause...

It's 10:30 in the morning on a rainy Thursday.

...pause...

How are you doing today?

Can I get you some fruit juice or water?"

... (perhaps gently hold her hand & smile)...

Known anniversaries (births, deaths, holidays, special memory dates) which may be nearing now include:

As nearly as I can tell, the date or time of day which seems to be their chosen time would be:

What time of day would *I* choose to die if that were something I had to choose right now?

Why?

*• I may like to choose the day and hour of my death...
What time is it now?*

Often there is a muddled confusion preceding death, when a semi-conscious person may be hovering between here and the Other Side and everything is confusing. One way you can help is to remind them who you are, what time it is, perhaps something about the day.

Also, if you have been openly discussing things like funeral or celebration arrangements, then you may want to try to be aware of any preferred day or time to die, (or not to die). This may be useful for you all. Some will say they want more people around when they die, so they do not want to die in the middle of the night. Others will say exactly the opposite because they *do not* want anyone around. And some will not care, or have not given it any thought.

If you do plan on asking these questions, be mindful of fatigue and the Breath Budget. Yes/No works best: Day? Night? Early? Late?, etc. Also try not to push.

Sometimes people are holding on for a special date or the arrival of someone specific from far away or even for news of an expected birth or death in the family.

Be mindful of anniversaries, special dates and friends or family who haven't yet come by to say goodbye. A better awareness of date and time can sometimes help your friend feel more at peace and in control.

How would I feel about being in their position and having someone touch me?

How do my own feelings about touch affect my tendency to touch now any more or any less?

In some cases where touch isn't appropriate or wasn't necessarily a part of your relationship, then we use personal space or proximity as a gauge:

Do I find myself chatting with them from a closer or further distance than normal?

Is this a conscious choice of mine?

Do I feel that their condition has affected my ability or desire to be in closer proximity?

• Touch me gently (but not distractingly) as I die. Be with me but do not demand that I be with you.

There is a special connectedness in the feel of touch. It helps to remind the dying person that they are still among the world of the living, still valued, still loved still treasured as the physical being they have always been.

It is, of course, necessary to be respectful of personal space and a sense of autonomy. There is a difference between *taking* in touch and *giving* in touch just as you yourself would realize in your own interactions. Best always to be mindful of appropriateness in touch, tending still those usual subtle messages.

In the case of AIDS and cancer, family members and friends can sometimes have unfounded and irrational fears of touching a dying person, as if a simple touch might somehow infect.

Somewhere is that gentle, supportive "middle ground" of appropriate genuine loving touch. Touch is important to us humans. It reinforces feelings of self-worth, value, love and kindness. It is a subtle, yet very real, communication of human acceptance, presence, respect and love, which a dying person still deserves to feel. (Try not to expect much touch in return right now, though, since strength could be at a premium at this point.)

Give your loving message through your loving touch.

Notes on apparent guides / visitors from the Other Side
which we have noticed here lately:
(Time / Date / Event / Those present)

Specific behaviors which seemed to indicate the
presence of a being or entity we may not have seen:

How do I feel about these things? Is there room in my
belief system to accept and understand?

• *Help me and encourage me to reach out and meet with the guides who may come to meet me.*

A large percentage of friends and family of persons nearing death report the presence of "visitors" or "guides" seemingly appearing to the dying person in an apparent willingness to assist in guiding them on their path to the Other Side or the After Life.

You may sometimes notice your loved one staring at the side or foot of the bed in a state of curiosity or intensity. Or they may reach out and mumble, whisper or speak with someone you cannot see. You may also notice a sudden feeling of peace and contentment come over them with either a wide-eyed stare or a retiring smile after they have been apparently reaching toward "someone who has come to visit."

Regardless of your own personal belief system in these matters, it is important that you remain as open-minded as possible. Try not to impose your beliefs, either to suggest they *must* reach out for visitors, or that they *must not* reach out for visitors. It is best to just try and be quietly supportive now, whatever their experience. If they feel your support and understanding, you may even hear some interesting stories about this time.

Trust in the love and support of guides
whom they trust and love.

(See also pages 74-77 in the "Beliefs" section.)

Specific last requests which I have heard about here and I want to be sure to remember:

What changes might I personally want to make in light of what I have learned during this process, so that my own last requests might be better taken care of?

Do I have a will yet?

• *My last requests are important to me.   Please assure me that you'll see that they're taken care of.*

If your friend or loved one is willing to speak openly about their impending death and certain arrangements they would like to make, or have you make, following their death, then count yourself fortunate.

You are being given a sort of homework assignment in grief. As you go through the process of planning and executing the points of their final requests, you are very likely to find yourself moving through the stages of grief more quickly, more fulfilled and more resolved.

In "being there" for your loved one at this time and in this capacity, you are helping to ease a strained feeling of helplessness on their part. And in being able to actually follow through with the requests, you are able to feel a sense of completion, devotion, commitment, love and respect.

Be happy you are able to be there.
Be at peace.

Fear, dread and overwhelm can be natural feelings as we attend a dying friend / loved one. But so can joy, compassion and tenderness. Realistically looking at both sides of the situation, then:

Things which have made it tough for me to be here:

1)

2)

3)

Yet things which have made me joyful I'm here:

1)

2)

3)

Important ways I expect to grow from having been here:

Who else do I know who should probably be encouraged to try and come by?

• *Please remember me as a Personal Being with history, and not just as the fragment you may find me to be now.*

One of the common dilemmas of friends, family and guests around the time of nearing death is an internal defensive monologue something like:

"Do I really need to go to see Aunt Millie? Why can't I just remember her as she was in my happy childhood memories?"

Perhaps the best way to answer this is merely to say that each of us has our personal history and beingness which is unique and everlasting. Yet each of us also has only one body in which we house that being, our temple where we receive physical visitors.

Encourage the visit. The children should be allowed and encouraged to visit, too, so that they can say their loving goodbyes. Like you, they will want to reinforce any wonderful loving memories. And they may be more ready to visit than you may think. Talking and sharing with children lovingly and sensitively now about life and death can be very helpful to them later in life.

Consider for a moment an ancient stone cathedral. We do not dishonor such a temple by a pilgrimage to it when it aches in ruin. Quite the contrary. Our lives are richer for the visit, having shared in love's journey.

Come. Visit your friend.
Allow, entrust your heart to lead.

Does this death process remind me of any others I've attended? How is it different? the same?

Am I aware of being nervous or impatient about the "destination" of this process or about something else?

If so, how might my nervousness affect us?

What kinds of things in life tend to make me impatient anyway? How might things here push my buttons?

How might I better relax and try to be more present?

• *Try to be patient and present in the process of these times. There is no schedule to the Hereafter.*

Death is an individual process and cannot be rehearsed in its entirety, no matter how many times one attends it. And yet certain aspects of the process can be better understood having had experience with the death of someone else.

There can be an impatience in this last period while waiting for "that time to come." It is like traveling along a lonely desert highway, signs promising this road leads somewhere.... There is a droning impatient knowingness that it is closer. Soon. Soon. Soon. Yet in between, an endless ribbon of days and hours and minutes where all we can do is go on waiting.

The death process will unfold in its inevitable course. In order to be present and available for our loved one, it is best that we strive to be as supportive and aware as possible, open to understanding each moment as it presents itself. Afterward, as we look back on the whole process together, it will seem more organized and understandable. In the moment by moment, though, it can often seem confused, scattered, and delayed.

For now, just try to be present. Trust in your ability to better see the Big Picture later.

Greater patience brings greater peace.
Understanding will come in time.

When I think in terms of loss now, some of the things
I will miss include:

1)

2)

3)

4)

And when I consider celebrating some of the gifts of
our relationship, some of what I can celebrate include:

1)

2)

3)

4)

Which of our stories brings me the greatest joy?

• *Celebrate my relationship with you when I'm gone,
rather than merely grieving its loss.*

It is normal when someone dies for us to feel a sense
of loss and grief. This is usually because we miss the
presence of the physical being. But there is so much
more to a relationship than just the physical being.

Memories are a significant part of the relationship, too,
which you will continue to carry with you even after
your friend or loved one is gone. And memories, like
stories, continue to endure for all of eternity, so long as
someone like you chooses to recall or tell them.

That is a great comfort. You have an opportunity, at
any time you wish, to rekindle these memories, share
them with others, or think about your lives together
and how you enriched each other.

As you consider now what is to come, take time to
consider the difference between focusing on loss, and
focusing on celebration of that abundant relationship.
Realize that memories and love are very real, and they
give you very real reason to celebrate whenever you
choose to remember.

Smile to have known Joy
with this Dear One before you.

Ways in which I realize this death has been for me a Teacher and a Reflector:

Things I'm learning (including things which I may not have expected to be learning just now):

• *Realize that I go before you now, at least in part, as Teacher and Reflector for where you one day will follow.*

Death is in many ways a teacher. But if death is a teacher, then many of us in the West don't seem to want to attend that lecture, to learn those lessons.

It is a good idea, however, to consider the possibility that since we find ourselves here now, this is a perfect opportunity to also commit to learn something about life and death. Certainly our own time will come.

There is a teaching in Chinese Taoism which says that in all darkness there is light, and in all light there is darkness. It is the black/white symbol of the yin-yang.

Most of us already clearly perceive the darkness in death. But the light? Twofold: As you are present and supportive now for your friend, so you are their light. And as they blaze that trail before you where you will one day follow, so they are yours.

It is both our responsibility and our joy for our light to shine in each other's darkness. It is a receptive appreciation and humility in our darkness which welcomes the light, streaming in from others. In death, then, there is also wisdom, if we are open to receiving it.

Do not dwell on the darkness of death.
Shine your light.

The strongest most poignant feeling which I have about
this death process right now is:

Three ways in which I feel this all has been a bit of a
Wake-Up Call for me:

1)

2)

3)

• *Know that I am the Present in an ongoing flow of Humanity in Motion.*

Certainly there exists in each of our lives a sense of continuity, something of a river of time flowing from the past, through us and our daily lives, and on into the mysterious veiled perplexity of the future.

The death of a cherished friend or loved one is one of those times in life where we have an almost unique opportunity to experience a sharp and distinct awareness of the present, as if frozen forever in time.

For the dying, though, there is little of that same kind of meaning in the word "future" and an almost equal emptiness in what we call "the past." Yet there is often still a distinct and powerful dynamic potency in this opportunity to know life from the "here and now."

This present moment is the force and the focus. It is everything. It is the fulcrum of eternity. Perhaps for us, this can be a wake-up call. Today! Here! Now!

As with a beautiful rose garden, yesterday there were seeds, tomorrow only thorns and soil. But Today, Here, Now: fragrant beautiful roses, delicate in their peace. And in their presence a beautiful promise and plea:

> This is *our* time.
> Be here now.

What feelings of fear, loss or abandonment am I experiencing?

How might I appropriately deal with these feelings?

What might I be holding onto which might keep me from being able to "grant permission" to let go now?

Can I truly say that I am ready to let go?

• *Don't try to hold onto me beyond my time. Don't keep my physical body here beyond its will.*

As your loved one proceeds toward death's door, there are appropriate times and letting-go points in the death process. And yet, there is a natural and understandable magnetic draw to life on the planet here as well.

A different kind of draw pulls toward death, in that the body processes are shutting down and making it more and more difficult for your loved one to continue to be here. One part of the letting-go process is their knowing that you, here on this side, have given them permission to let go, permission to do what they need to do now. Have you?

It is important that you be able to work through your own fears of letting go, your attachments and your grudges, your hesitation and your worries. You need to get to the point where you can honestly and presently be there for your friend, supportive of their need now to let go and move on over to that Other Side.

> Letting go isn't saying "Goodbye."
> It's saying "Thank you."

I will always have my memories. Knowing that, I can more easily let go. Five memories which I can hold onto even after I let go:

1)

2)

3)

4)

5)

• *Seek to release your attachment to my body as you deepen your relationship to what we meant to one another in life.*

Some friends and family may have trouble realizing the difference between the body and the being; the physical person and the personality; the history and the memories. But it is important to be able to make these distinctions.

In order for your loved one now to more comfortably get on with the matter of releasing ties to the physical body and shutting on down, it may be necessary for some friends and family to directly or indirectly give permission to die.

If you feel that you and/or friends or family members may be still holding onto your friend or loved one, it might be a good idea to talk with each other to help encourage releasing attachment to the body. Giving permission to die can be silent or aloud, depending on what feels right in your circumstance.

Be present in the moment. Breathe deeply.

Know that memories never die.
Feel the feelings deep within you still.
Love always.

How might my beliefs of Eternity, Hereafter or stories of passage help to better illustrate our connection?

How does my friend / loved one's version of Eternity seem like my own, or differ from my own?

Other than my own view of things, how else might someone choose to see the interconnectedness of life?

• Help me to be aware of that grand stream of spirit, light, and consciousness.

According to most religions and spiritual teachings, a dying person is often met on the Other Side by friends and family members who have gone before, who help them to move into a lightness of being, and away from the heaviness of this physical body's passing.

A dying person may feel a weakening connection to the living and a stronger connection to friends and family who have gone before. They may also speak of a diffuse connection to Eternity, Heaven or the entire Universe itself where all things unite. But because it can be so disorienting, this "multiple awareness" can also be fearful or confusing to those who may not be ready to see it.

You can help now with a reminder that you support their safe passage to the Other Side. Help encourage them to recognize and connect with whatever religious or spiritual beings their belief system might suggest, such as guides, angels, Jesus, Buddha, Mohammed, or past friends and family who have gone before.

Quietly sharing spiritual songs, prayers and stories of the eternal hereafter (if consistent with your friend's beliefs) can help bring greater peace of mind to you both.

Help them find love and peace
as you share your peace and love.

What greater bonds have we shared, since I have been able to be here during this time?

What am I feeling about how all of this affects me?

What gave me strength to be here?

• *Give some thought to what you're going through right now. Has your being with me been helpful and healing for you as well?*

It is important that you know how much it means to your loved one that you have chosen to be here. This has not been an easy ordeal for anyone, not the person on the bed, and not for persons such as yourself who have been able to be here to help during the process.

Please take a moment now to reflect on this:
   You did not have to be here. You chose to be here, and that has made all of the difference.

Perhaps it is time to think a bit about how you are feeling. Consider how all of this is affecting you and your ability to continue to process your own understanding of priorities, love, resolution and that whole host of your own emotional and spiritual issues.

Remember that your feelings are an equally important part of this overall process, too.

Thank You for being here now.
Thank you for taking the risk to be present.

What specific actions can I take to help to make the world a better place in my understanding of this death process?

Can I think of a particular person, project or group who might benefit from my time or experience?

• *Help improve understanding in the world through your understanding of my death process.*

There is a great deal of misunderstanding in the world and it does seem that, for many people, the process of death and dying adds even more. Perhaps now is a good time, however, to choose to begin to clear up some of that misunderstanding by taking appropriate action.

Many people report a profound shift in their life view following the process surrounding the death of a close friend or relative. There is often a positive shift in awareness which occurs, allowing and encouraging them to reach out again, this time to help someone else involved in the turmoil of the death process.

If you feel as a result of your own process here that you might have a bit of available energy, resources or time to contribute to others, then there is no doubt a place for it. There will always be plenty of hospices, hospitals and outreach programs who would love to work with whatever energy you can offer now.

Every family, every friend, of
someone at the end of life
is a person in need.

Reviewing the list on the facing page, what I feel about seeing these symptoms is:

Who might answer any questions I have?

What clarification questions do I have about certain items on the list? Do I understand what each means?

Observations / Notes on the end-stage process:

• *There is a pattern to the body's shutting down process. Your familiarity with the process will help.*

Though some persons may not exhibit all symptoms, or may exhibit them in a different order, these are the most common end-stage symptoms to be aware of:

• General disorientation and confusion of time, space, relation to visitors or even to who or where self is.
• Marked increase in agitation; fear of abandonment.
• Pulling, picking, grasping at clothing, bedclothes; may react with panic to bedding too loose or too tight.
• Staring off toward, or reaching out for, someone not physically present whom they seem to see.
• Conscious hours decline, sleeping almost all the time.
• Almost total loss of appetite, hunger and thirst.
• Uneven and irregular breathing and heartbeat.
• Breathing rate which increases and decreases, even stops altogether for 5-50 seconds, then starts again with deep sudden gasp. [Cheyne-Stokes breathing]
• Yellowing, loss of coloration in face and general body.
• Speckled, deepened mottled coloration of limbs and extremities, also cool or clammy to the touch.
• Loss of control of bowel and bladder. [incontinence]
• Significant increase in mucous in mouth and throat.
• Strained, altered, labored breathing. [the death rattle]

Please realize that it is normal to feel overwhelmed with discomfort reading through these symptoms. They are provided here only that you may be better informed of the pattern and the process. You may wish to consult the list in reference from time to time.

In the last few hours or couple days, what particular rallies or change in state of mind have I noticed?

Has there been a change in awareness or behavior, or any particular sense of knowingness and acceptance?

How have these last few hours / days' process seemed to me? Peaceful? Different? Does this seem like it might be the beginning of the "end-stage" process?

• *Satottà toki ga shinu toki.* — JAPANESE PROVERB
The time of death is a time of knowingness.

It is difficult to know exactly when the "end-stage" process actually begins to occur. But often as death approaches there is a profound and silent knowingness which comes over a dying person as if a sense of peace and acceptance were poured into that fragile frame. It may be marked by a kind of unexpected rally first.

From that point forward it is usually no more than a few days until death. The struggle is no more, and with this resolution usually comes a calm and gentle serenity which gradually diminishes into death. There is less challenge, less struggle, less pain now. There is less concern about separating from life and the living.

What might have before been perceived as alienation and loss seems now to be seen from the Other Side, from the vantage point of belonging and release, of love and peace. All grows still.

Death can sometimes seem to us both terrible beauty and bewildering awe, its demanding forthright process an inescapable call. And yet when all is still and knowingness finds its peace, what is that call, but a call to serenity, to rest, to memory and release?

Trust that your loved one will know Peace.
Open to trust.

Notes on the final bedside vigil group present:
(though you may want to come back and fill this out later after a few days or hours have passed)

Who was present during the final hours / moments of death, what was the situation and how did it unfold?

What can we do / did we do to make sure that these final few hours are peaceful and gently supportive?

• Be calm as I die— in those final moments— and allow the current of spirit to carry me away gently, gradually.

Some religious and spiritual teachings suggest that the final moments of life are the most important of all of life itself, that it is the resolution and passage of this stage which ultimately determines this being's placement in eternity.

Regardless of your own personal beliefs, it remains a respectful and compassionate act of loving kindness to honor a person's quiet passage in these final moments.

In this quiet calmness, now is the time to continue to verbally offer your loved one assurances of your love, support, and well-being. It is very likely they can still hear the reassuring sound of your voice, whether they seem conscious at this point or not.

Hold a hand. Share appropriate prayers or messages consistent with their belief system. Remind them that you are present and available, that you support their reaching out now for the lightness of being on the Other Side. Let them know that they can leave behind the distressed and burdened body now, that you will look after it, and that you will be okay. Wish them well on their journey. Bid them peace and love and thanks.

These final moments
can be beautiful moments of release.

Date / Time of Death:

List of persons present at time of death:

What were my reactions as it took place?

How did the moment unfold?

How do I feel now that it's all over?

• What a relief to leave that broken, burdened body behind. It is difficult to go, yes, but what a relief at the same time. Thank You so much for your help.

There is often a mingling of sadness and relief when it is all over. Your loved one was finally able to let go, released from the pain and discomfort of the physical body. And yet: it is indeed all over.

They *did* let go. They *did* depart. Left now
a shell, an empty cocoon, a mask, a gown.
But soul, it is clear, has gone.

This most intense concern of yours for these last few days, weeks or months now draws to a close. It is time to let other concerns back into your life again.

These can be bittersweet moments. Certainly you are relieved that your loved one is no longer suffering, yet your own pain of the loss may linger closely still. Trust that this, too, shall pass.

These are solemn moments: quiet, lonely footsteps on a sacred path. In this silence begins a new journey for you both.

For your loved one: Eternity.
And for you: the Way Back.

All of Life awaits your next breath.
Breathe deeply.

Notes on our Closing Ritual and/or Prayers for this time:

The process of what we chose to do in the minutes and hours immediately following death was...

Sample Closing Rituals before the body is taken away: Some people will have a ritual preparation and washing of the body. Some sit with the body and reminisce or sing together. Some choose to write poetry, or short memorials. Some take photographs of the final vigil group together (with the body or not). Some have a banquet. Some have a prayer circle or religious service (at the bedside or a chapel). Some merely choose to sit quietly with the body and think, or write or pray.

You may choose to do none, some or all of these. Any closing ritual is always a personal choice of friends and family present.

• Do not disturb my body as it reclines afterward. Give it at least a few minutes to a few hours' respite.

With respect for cultural and spiritual perspectives, it is a good idea to allow the body to recline in peace for a time after death. This gives the newly departed being an opportunity to gently and gradually move forward in comfortable confidence to the Other Side. Surely in most cases there is no need to move the body yet, and especially when your loved one's spiritual beliefs might propose such a waiting period, it is best to honor this principle and tradition.

It is not uncommon in many traditions for next-of-kin, or those in special bond with the departed being, to continue sitting vigil with the body for a period. This allows for maintaining a quiet link of community a bit longer, as soul's venue changes over to the spiritual plane, and the body's temple receives its final visitors.

This is usually a time of prayer, spiritual guidance and accompanying contemplation, reminders to the loved one that they have moved on, beyond their pain in this life, toward peace as their new journey begins.

You may wish at this time to observe your personal closing ritual if you have one prepared.

Farewell, my friend, we thank you for your gift
of love and friendship in our lives. A full
emboldened breath we breathe now sighs "Farewell!"

Any final reflections on this disease / cause of death?

What are the three most important things I have learned during this process:

1)

2)

3)

How has this taught me more about love?

• Maybe AIDS and cancer aren't just the scourges and the detestable diseases we've often thought them to be. Maybe they were put on the planet to teach people about Love.
— overheard in a hospice break room, 3:30 a.m.

It is said that we often learn most from our greatest challenges in life. And one of the surest ways for us to begin to understand and experience love is to selflessly share it with others.

Interestingly enough, the experience of choosing to be a caregiver for a friend or loved one at the end of life often combines these two opportunities into one.

The challenge of being present for a friend or loved one at the end of life reminds us of life's priorities, its patterns, and what is asked of us in the process.

If you think back to when you first heard of your friend or loved one's diagnosis and how you thought about it at the time, did you then understand what was about to happen? Did you realize this experience could be such an abundant gift of learning, growing and sharing?

How has this experience changed how you see life and death or how you see this illness?

Sometimes Love has a strange way of finding us.

URGENT
WHISPERS
CARE OF THE DYING
Afterword

Now that this process is drawing to a close, you have had an opportunity to work with and complete at least some of the material and exercises in the book. I hope these materials have been useful for you to anticipate some of your loved one's needs and process, as well as how you might better understand and respond to them.

Now it is time to turn attention back to your own path, to family, life, priorities. Most people at this time begin to slow down a bit, retreating and seeking to regroup and concentrate more on a kind of healing. That may involve a personal voyage inward, thinking and pondering about some of what you've been through. Or it may involve a more outward process where you participate with friends, family or community members in shared activities of some kind.

Whatever your choice, it is appropriate to begin thinking about how you will be dealing with some of your feelings of grief. Personal coping and grieving rituals take many different forms. Try to tap into or develop one of your own which is both meaningful and useful for you.

If you were able to take the time to do some of the exercises in the book and have collected notes of some of the events and your thoughts and feelings along the way, then perhaps now would be a good time to begin to take a look at some of those. Just going over them will be helpful to you as you think about moving forward.

If you were fortunate enough to be able to go through this process with friends or family, or if you were able to meet new friends along the way, then you may want to spend some time together talking about things. You can compare notes, talk about your experiences, share some of what each of you may have thought about or written about in the exercise sections if you did them. Sharing these stories and experiences can be therapeutic for you both as you move on and grow.

No doubt you better understand now what it means to Learn, Grow and Share, having experienced this remarkable journey with your friend or loved one. Although this was a process around death and dying, you probably also better understand the preciousness of life and living now, and how just being present for a friend or loved one in their final days can be such a rewarding comfort, bringing gifts of Spirit to you both. Thank You for taking the time to be here and share your path of personal discovery as you tuned in to be present for your loved one's ***Urgent Whispers***.

-JS

Notes:

Your comments are welcome about the usefulness of this book for your purpose. Feel free to write to the address in the front of the book or email: Whispers@Bardo.ORG You may also wish to visit the Urgent Whispers web site at the Bardo of Death Studies: http://WWW.Bardo.ORG/UW/

*If you enjoyed **Urgent Whispers: Care of the Dying**, you may want to check with your bookseller for other titles available from L L X Press in the **Urgent Whispers** line.*

ASHES TO ASHES
AND DUST TO DUST
SO AS WITH TIME
SO HERE WE MUST

RELEASE THE TIES
THE BONDS SET FREE
THAT FRIENDS MIGHT FIND
ETERNITY.

*-from "Farewell, Scott" a poem for the
scattering of ashes of friend Scott Lucas
Multnomah Falls, Oregon, 3/3/95
- Jerral Sapienza*

URGENT WHISPERS

CARE OF THE DYING

Topical Index

A

B

H

I

J

K

L

Y

NOTES:

URGENT
WHISPERS
CARE OF THE DYING
Technical Notes

The manuscript was originally written longhand over several years and several hundred hours sitting vigil, pondering and composing in Portland, Eugene and Newport, Oregon; Seattle, Washington; San Francisco and Truckee, California; Arlington Heights and Chicago, Illinois; Stuttgart, Germany and Scheffau, Austria and sometimes on trains and planes between these and other cities, interspersed with coffeehouse visits for relaxation and edit session time.

Initial digital input was via my notebook computers using Corel WordPerfect flowed into Adobe PageMaker where final edits were then transferred to digital masters and forwarded to our printer. Except for our reader spreads, the manuscript and "paste-up" never saw paper between input and digital output!

Main book typeface is 11.5pt Times New Roman; intro is in 12pt; this is in 9pt. 12-15pt Chevara is the interesting font for Vigil Notes and Closing Poem; 18pt Futura Light for the section headers on 10% screens, which incidentally were imported from Adobe PhotoShop based on the cover title font.

Book concept and design by Jerral Sapienza. Early eagle eye proofs by Fern Sapienza, Lynn Olsen, Teri Everden. Editing and proofing by Jerral Sapienza and Holly Saunders. Indexing review by Nancy Radius of Indexing Works. Printing, binding and production management by Tom Creamer of ProGraphics Services. What a great team to be working with!

Incidentally, the production team is also deeply indebted to Al Gore for inventing the Internet :-) which allowed writer, artists, editors and reviewers to collaborate across several time zones!

To order additional copies of this book, photocopy this page and take it to your local bookseller or send a check or money order in US Dollars to:

L L X Press
Book Orders
PO Box 380
Eugene, OR 97440-0380 =USA=

Urgent Whispers: Care of the Dying by **Jerral Sapienza** is available in two distinct binding formats. Please specify how many of each binding format you wish to order.

Qty:	Description	Price	Extension
	ISBN: **0-9717107-0-8**		
_____	Standard Paperback Edition		
	4¼" x 7", 152 pp	US **$14.95**	_____
	ISBN: **0-9717107-5-9**		
_____	Coil Bound (Spiral) Edition		
	4¼" x 7", 152 pp	US **$14.95**	_____

Shipping / Handling for all US Addresses:
$3.00 first book; $2.00 each additional book
Overseas: $9.00 first book; $5.00 ea additional   _____

Order Total in US Funds $ _____

In case we have questions about your order:

Phone ( ) _____

Email: _____

Ship to: _____

_____

_____

_____

CAN YOU
DRINK
THE CUP?

HENRI J.M. NOUWEN

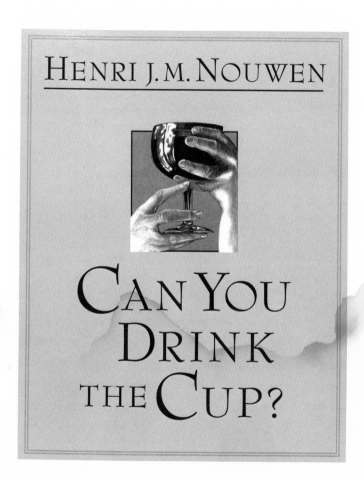

CAN YOU
DRINK
THE CUP?

AVE MARIA PRESS   Notre Dame, Indiana 46556

International Standard Book Number: 0-87793-581-5
0-87793-582-3 (CB)

Illustrations by Jane Pitz

Cover design by Elizabeth J. French

Printed and bound in the United States of America.

Library of Congress Cataloging-in-Publication Data

Nouwen, Henri J. M.
     Can you drink the cup? / Henri J. M. Nouwen.
          p.   cm.
     ISBN 0-87793-582-3 (cloth). — ISBN 0-87793-581-5 (paper)
     1. Spiritual life—Catholic Church. 2. Nouwen, Henri J. M.
I. Title.
BX2350.2.N6695   1996
248.4′82—dc20   96-24924
                                                               CIP

In Memory of

Adam John Arnett

November 17, 1961 — February 13, 1996

Acknowledgments

This little book was written during the first few months of my sabbatical year, a year that the l'Arche Daybreak community gave me for my writing. I am deeply grateful to all the members of the community, and especially to Nathan Ball, the director, and Sue Mosteller, the pastor, for their encouragement and support during this time away from home.

I also owe much gratitude to Peggy McDonnell, her family and friends who, in memory of Murray McDonnell, offered me the financial support for my writing.

I wrote *Can You Drink the Cup?* while staying with Hans and Margaret Kruitwagen in Oakville, Ontario, and with Robert Jonas, Margaret Bullitt-Jonas, and their son, Sam, in Watertown, Massachusetts. Their great kindness and generous hospitality offered me the ideal context for reflection and writing. A special word of thanks goes to Margaret Bullitt-Jonas's mother, Sarah Doering, who offered me the use of her third-floor apartment while she made a three-month Buddhist retreat.

I am also most grateful to Kathy Christie for her very competent and efficient secretarial help and for her great patience with my many "urgent" calls and "important" changes of mind. Her friendship is a real gift to me. A special word of thanks goes to Susan Brown, whose last minute line-editing was an unexpected blessing, and to Wendy Greer, who made many valuable corrections.

Finally, I want to thank my editor Frank Cunningham at Ave Maria Press for his long-term interest in my writing and his special care for the presentation of this text.

I dedicate *Can You Drink the Cup?* to Adam Arnett, my friend and teacher about whom I wrote in these pages. Adam died on February 13, 1996 just at the time this text was finished. I hope and pray that his life and death will continue to bear much fruit in the lives of all those who have known him and loved him so much.

Contents

Then the mother of Zebedee's sons came with her sons to make a request of Jesus and bowed low; and he said to her, "What is it that you want?" She said to him, "Promise that these two sons of mine may sit one at your right hand and the other at your left in your kingdom." Jesus answered, "You do not know what you are asking. Can you drink the cup that I am going to drink?" They replied, "We can." He said to them, "Very well; you shall drink my cup, but as for seats at my right hand and my left, these are not mine to grant; they belong to those to whom they have been allotted by my Father."

(Matthew 20:20-23)

THE CHALICE AND THE CUP

It was Sunday, July 21, 1957. Bernard Alfrink, the Cardinal Archbishop of the Netherlands, laid his hands on my head, dressed me with a white chasuble, and offered me his golden chalice to touch with my hands bound together with a linen cloth. Thus, along with twenty-seven other candidates, I was ordained to the priesthood in St. Catherine's Cathedral in Utrecht. I will never forget the deep emotions that stirred my heart at that moment.

Since I was six years old, I had felt a great desire to be a priest. Except for a few fleeting thoughts of becoming a navy captain, mostly because of the influence of the men with their blue and white uniforms and golden stripes parading the railroad platform of our town, I always dreamt about one day being able to say Mass, as my uncle Anton did.

My maternal grandmother was my great supporter. An astute businesswoman, she had built a large department store, where my mother did some part-time bookkeeping work and where I could run around, use the elevators freely, and play hide-and-seek with my younger brother. As soon as she discovered my budding vocation to the priesthood, she ordered her store carpenter to build me a child-size altar and had her seamstress sew all the vestments necessary to play priest. By the time I was eight years old, I had converted the attic of our home to a children's chapel, where I played Mass, gave sermons to my parents and relatives, and set up a whole hierarchy with bishops, priests, deacons, and altar servers among my friends. Meanwhile, my grandmother not only continued to give me new things to play priest with, such as chalices and plates, but also gently introduced me to a life of prayer and encouraged me in a personal relationship with Jesus.

When I was twelve years old I wanted to go the minor seminary, but both my parents felt that I was much too young to leave home. "You are not ready to make a decision about the priesthood," my father told me. "You better wait until you are eighteen." It was 1944, and they wanted me to go to a gymnasium in our town, close to Amsterdam. The Second

World War had come to a very critical stage, but my parents were able to keep me and my brother away from the cruelties of war and even provided us with a rather regular school life. After the war we moved to The Hague, where I finished my secondary education. Finally, in 1950, I went to the seminary to study philosophy and theology and prepare myself for ordination.

On that 21st day of July, 1957, when my life-long dream to become a priest was realized, I was a very naive twenty-five-year-old. My life had been well-protected. I had grown up as in a beautifully kept garden surrounded by thick hedges. It was a garden of loving parental care, innocent boy scout experiences, daily mass and communion, long hours of study with very patient teachers, and many years of happy but very isolated seminary life. I came out of it all full of love for Jesus, and full of desire to bring the Gospel to the world, but without being fully aware that not everybody was waiting for me. I had only met—and that quite cautiously—a few Protestants, had never encountered an unbeliever, and certainly had no idea about other religions. Divorced people were unknown to me, and if there were any priests who had left the priesthood, they were kept away from me. The greatest "scandal" I had experienced was a friend leaving the seminary!

Still, life in the garden of my youth was quite beautiful and offered me invaluable gifts for the rest of my life: a joyful spirit, a deep devotion for Jesus and Mary, a true desire to pray, a great love for theology and spirituality, a good knowledge of contemporary languages, a serious interest in scripture and the early Christian writers, an enthusiasm about preaching, and a very strong sense of vocation. My maternal grandmother, my paternal grandparents, my parents, friends, and teachers all encouraged me to trust my desire to live a life with Jesus for others.

When Cardinal Alfrink handed me the chalice, I felt ready to start a life as a priest. The joy of that day still lives in me as a precious memory. The chalice was the sign of that joy.

Most of my classmates had chalices made for their ordination. I was an exception. My uncle Anton, who was ordained in 1922, offered me his chalice as a sign of his gratitude that a new priest had come into our family. It was beautiful, made by a famous Dutch goldsmith and adorned with my grandmother's diamonds. The foot was decorated with a crucifix shaped as a tree of life, from which golden grapes and grape leaves grew to cover the node and bowl. Around the rim of the foot these Latin words were engraved: *"Ego sum vites, vos palmites,"* which means, "I am the vine, you are the branches." It was a very precious gift, and I was deeply moved to receive it. I remember saying to my uncle: "I have seen you celebrating Mass so often with this chalice; can you really do without it?" He smiled and said, "I want you to have it. It comes from your grandmother, who died too soon to see you as a priest but whose love for you, her oldest grandchild, is with you today." When I still hesitated to accept the chalice, he said: "Take it, but pass it on to the next member of our family who will be ordained."

The chalice is still with me, because so far no one else in my family has been ordained to the priesthood. I keep it in the sacristy of the Dayspring Chapel in Toronto, where I now live. I often show it to friends and visitors. But so much has happened during the thirty-seven years that followed my ordination that my uncle's decorated golden chalice no longer expresses what I am presently living. During the Eucharist today, I use several large cups made by the glassblower Simon Pearce in Vermont. The precious golden chalice that could only be touched and used by an ordained priest is replaced by large glass cups in which the wine can be seen and from which many can drink. These glass cups speak about a new way of being a priest and a new way of being human. I am happy with these cups on the altar table today, but without the golden chalice given me by my uncle Anton nearly forty years ago, they would not mean as much to me as they do.

Introduction

THE QUESTION

In this book I want to tell the story of the cup, not just as my story, but as the story of life.

When Jesus asks his friends James and John, the sons of Zebedee, "Can you drink the cup that I am going to drink?" he poses the question that goes right to the heart of my priesthood and my life as a human being. Years ago, when I held that beautiful golden chalice in my hands, that question didn't seem hard to answer. For me, a newly ordained priest full of ideas and ideals, life seemed to be rich with promises. I was eager to drink the cup!

Today, sitting in front of a low table surrounded by men and women with mental disabilities and their assistants, and offering them the glass cups of wine, that same question has

19

become a spiritual challenge. Can I, can we, drink the cup that Jesus drank?

I still remember the day, a few years ago, when the story in which Jesus raises that question was read during the Eucharist. It was 8:30 in the morning, and about twenty members of the Daybreak community were gathered in the little basement chapel. Suddenly the words "Can you drink the cup?" pierced my heart like the sharp spear of a hunter. I knew at that moment—as with a flash of insight—that taking this question seriously would radically change our lives. It is the question that has the power to crack open a hardened heart and lay bare the tendons of the spiritual life.

"Can you drink the cup? Can you empty it to the dregs? Can you taste all the sorrows and joys? Can you live your life to the full whatever it will bring?" I realized these were our questions.

But why should we drink this cup? There is so much pain, so much anguish, so much violence. Why should we drink the cup? Wouldn't it be a lot easier to live normal lives with a minimum of pain and a maximum of pleasure?

After the reading, I spontaneously grabbed one of the large glass cups standing on the table in front of me and looking at those around me—some of whom could hardly walk, speak, hear, or see—I said: "Can we hold the cup of life in our hands?

Can we lift it up for others to see, and can we drink it to the full?" Drinking the cup is much more than gulping down whatever happens to be in there, just as breaking the bread is much more than tearing a loaf apart. Drinking the cup of life involves *holding, lifting,* and *drinking.* It is the full celebration of being human.

Can we hold our life, lift our life, and drink it, as Jesus did? In some of those around me, there was a sign of recognition, but in myself there was a deep awareness of truth. Jesus' question had given me a new language with which to speak about my life and the lives of those around me. For a long time after that simple morning Eucharist, I kept hearing Jesus' question: "Can you drink the cup that I am going to drink?" Just letting that question sink in made me feel very uncomfortable. But I knew that I had to start living with it.

This book is the fruit of having done that. It strives to make Jesus' question pierce our hearts so that a personal answer can emerge from there. I will follow the three themes that emerged that morning in the Dayspring Chapel: *holding, lifting,* and *drinking.* They will allow me to explore the spiritual horizons that Jesus' question opens for us and to invite you who will read this to join me in this exploration.

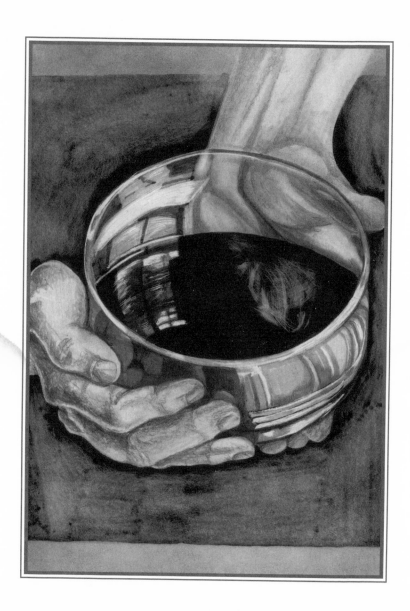

Part 1

HOLDING
THE CUP

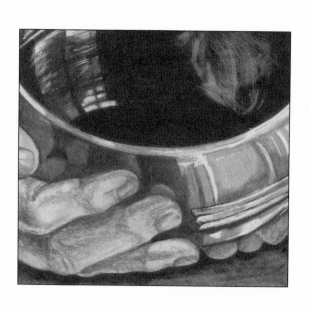

Chapter 1

HOLDING

Before we drink the cup, we must hold it!

I still remember a family dinner long ago in the Netherlands. It was a special occasion, but I have forgotten whether it was a birthday, a wedding, or an anniversary. Since I was still a young boy, I was not allowed to drink wine, but I was fascinated by the way the grown-ups were drinking their wine! After the wine had been poured into the glasses, my uncle took his glass, put both of his hands around the cup, moved the glass gently while letting the aroma enter his nostrils, looked at all the people around the table, lifted it up, took a little sip, and said: "Very good . . . a very good wine . . . let me see the bottle . . . it must be a fiftier."

This was my uncle Anton, my mother's oldest brother, priest, monsignor, authority in many things, good wines being one of them. Every time uncle Anton came to family dinners, he had a comment or two to make about the wine that was served. He would say, "A full body," or "Not what I expected," or "Could be a little hardier," or "This is just good with the roast," or "Well, for fish this is okay." His criticisms were not always appreciated by my father, who provided the wine, but nobody dared to contradict him. The whole ritual around the wine intrigued me as a child. Often my brothers and I would tease our uncle, saying: "Well, uncle Anton, can you guess the year this wine was made without looking at the label? You are the expert, aren't you?"

One thing I learned from it all: drinking wine is more than just drinking. You have to know what you are drinking, and you have to be able to talk about it. Similarly, just living life is not enough. We must know what we are living. A life that is not reflected upon isn't worth living. It belongs to the essence of being human that we contemplate our life, think about it, discuss it, evaluate it, and form opinions about it. Half of living is reflecting on what is being lived. Is it worth it? Is it good? Is it bad? Is it old? Is it new? What is it all about? The greatest joy as well as the greatest pain of living come not only from what we live but even more from how we think and feel about what we are living. Poverty and wealth, success and failure, beauty and ugliness aren't just the facts of life. They are realities that are lived very differently by different people, depending on the way they are placed in the larger scheme of things. A poor person who has compared his poverty with the wealth of his neighbor and thought about the discrepancy lives his poverty very differently than the person who has no wealthy neighbor and has never been able to make a comparison. Reflection is essential for growth, development, and change. It is the unique power of the human person.

Holding the cup of life means looking critically at what we are living. This requires great courage, because when we start looking, we might be terrified by what we see. Questions may arise that we don't know how to answer. Doubts may come up about things we thought we were sure about. Fear may emerge from unexpected places. We are tempted to say: "Let's just live life. All this thinking about it only makes things harder." Still, we intuitively know that without looking at life critically we lose our vision and our direction. When we drink the cup without holding it first, we may simply get drunk and wander around aimlessly.

Holding the cup of life is a hard discipline. We are thirsty people who like to start drinking at once. But we need to restrain our impulse to drink, put both of our hands around the cup, and ask ourselves, "What am I given to drink? What is in my cup? Is it safe to drink? Is it good for me? Will it bring me health?"

Just as there are countless varieties of wine, there are countless varieties of lives. No two lives are the same. We often compare our lives with those of others, trying to decide whether we are better or worse off, but such comparisons do not help us much. We have to live our life, not someone else's. We have to hold *our own* cup. We have to dare to say: "This is my life, the life that is given to me, and it is this life that I have to live, as well as I can. My life is unique. Nobody else will ever live it. I have my own history, my own family, my own body, my own character, my own friends, my own way of thinking, speaking, and acting—yes, I have my own life to live. No one else has the same challenge. I am alone, because I am unique. Many people can help me to live my life, but after all is said and done, I have to make my own choices about how to live."

It is hard to say this to ourselves, because doing so confronts us with our radical aloneness. But it is also a wonderful challenge, because it acknowledges our radical uniqueness.

I am reminded of Philip Sears's powerful sculpture of Pumunangwet, the Native American at the Fruitlands Museums in Harvard, Massachusetts. He stands with his beautifully stretched naked body, girded with a loincloth, reaching to the heavens with his bow high above him in his left hand while his right hand still holds the memory of the arrow that just left for the stars. He is totally self-possessed, solidly rooted on the earth, and totally free to aim far beyond himself. He knows who he is. He is proud to be a lonesome warrior called to fulfill a sacred task. He truly holds his own.

Like that warrior we must hold our cup and fully claim who we are and what we are called to live. Then we too can shoot for the stars!

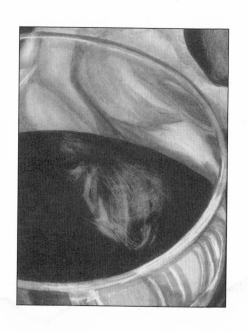

Chapter 2

THE CUP OF SORROW

When I first came to l'Arche Daybreak, I saw much sorrow.

I was asked to care for Adam, a twenty-two-year-old man who could not speak, could not walk alone, did not show signs of recognition. He had a curved back, suffered from daily epileptic seizures, and often had intestinal pains. When I first met Adam, I was afraid of him. His many handicaps made him a stranger to me, a man I wanted to avoid.

Soon after I met Adam I also came to know his brother Michael. Although Michael could speak a little and was able to walk by himself and even fulfill some minor tasks, he too was severely handicapped and needed constant attention to make it through the day. Adam and Michael are the only children of Jeanne and Rex.

Michael lived at home until he was twenty-five and Adam until he was eighteen. Jeanne and Rex would have loved to continue to keep the boys at home. However, time was eroding the physical resources required to look after their sons and so they entrusted them to the l'Arche Daybreak community, hoping to find a good home for them there.

I was quite overwhelmed with the sorrows of this little family. Four people burdened by worries and pain, by fear of unexpected complications, by the inability to communicate clearly, by a sense of great responsibility, and by an awareness that life will only become harder as age increases.

But Adam, Michael, and their parents are part of a much greater sorrow. There is Bill, who suffers from muscular dystrophy, who needs a pacemaker for his heart and a breathing machine for his lungs during the night, and who is in constant fear of falling. He has no parents to visit. His parents never were able to care for him, and both died at a rather young age.

There is Tracy, completely paralyzed, but with a bright mind, always struggling to find ways to express her feelings and thoughts. There is Susanne, not only mentally disabled but also regularly battered by inner voices that she cannot control. There is Loretta, whose disability causes her to feel unwanted by family and friends and whose search for affection and affirmation throws her into moments of deep despair and depression. There are David, Francis, Patrick, Janice, Carol, Gordie, George, Patsy . . . each of them with a cup full of sorrow.

Surrounding them are men and women of different ages, from different countries and religions, trying to assist these wounded people. But they soon discover that those they care for reveal to them their own less visible but no less real sorrows: sorrows about broken families, sexual unfulfillment, spiritual alienation, career doubts, and most of all, confusing relationships. The more they look at their own often wounded pasts and confront their uncertain futures, the more they see how much sorrow there is in their lives.

And for me things are not very different. After ten years of living with people with mental disabilities and their assistants, I have become deeply aware of my own sorrow-filled heart. There was a time when I said: "Next year I will finally have it together," or "When I grow more mature these moments of inner darkness will go," or "Age will diminish my emotional needs." But now I know that my sorrows are mine and will not leave me. In fact I know they are very old and very deep sorrows, and that no amount of positive thinking or optimism will make them less. The adolescent struggle to find someone to love me is still there; unfulfilled needs for affirmation as a young adult remain alive in me. The deaths of my mother and many family members and friends during my later years cause me continual grief. Beyond all that, I experience deep sorrow that I have not become who I wanted to be, and that the God to whom I have prayed so much has not given me what I have most desired.

But what is our sorrow in a little community in Canada, compared with the sorrow of the city, the country, and the world? What about the sorrow of the homeless people asking for money on the streets of Toronto, what about the young men and women dying of AIDS, what about the thousands who live in prisons, mental hospitals, and nursing homes? What about the broken families, the unemployed, and the countless disabled men and women who have no safe place such as Daybreak?

And when I look beyond the boundaries of my own city and country, the picture of sorrow becomes even more frightening. I see parentless children roaming the streets of São Paulo like packs of wolves. I see young boys and girls being sold as prostitutes in Bangkok. I see the emaciated prisoners of war in the camps of former Yugoslavia. I see the naked bodies of people in Ethiopia and Somalia wandering aimlessly in the eroded desert. I see millions of lonely, starving faces all over the world, and large piles of the dead bodies of people killed in cruel wars and ethnic conflicts. Whose cup is this? It is our cup, the cup of human suffering. For each of us our sorrows are deeply personal. For all of us our sorrows, too, are universal.

Now I look at the man of sorrows. He hangs on a cross with outstretched arms. It is Jesus, condemned by Pontius Pilate, crucified by Roman soldiers, and ridiculed by Jews and Gentiles alike. But it is also us, the whole human race, people of all times and all places, uprooted from the earth as a spectacle of agony for the entire universe to watch. "When I am lifted up from the earth," Jesus said, "I shall draw all people to myself" (John 12:32). Jesus, the man of sorrows, and we, the people of sorrow, hang there between heaven and earth, crying out, "God, our God, why have you forsaken us?"

"Can you drink the cup that I am going to drink?" Jesus asked his friends. They answered yes, but had no idea what he was talking about. Jesus' cup is the cup of sorrow, not just his own sorrow but the sorrow of the whole human race. It is a cup full of physical, mental, and spiritual anguish. It is the cup of starvation, torture, loneliness, rejection, abandonment, and immense anguish. It is the cup full of bitterness. Who wants to drink it? It is the cup that Isaiah calls "the cup of God's wrath. The chalice, the stupefying cup, you have drained to the dregs," (Isaiah 51:17) and what the second angel in the

Book of Revelation calls "the wine of retribution" (Revelation 14:8), which Babylon gave the whole world to drink.

When the moment to drink that cup came for Jesus, he said: "My soul is sorrowful to the point of death" (Matthew 26:38). His agony was so intense that "his sweat fell to the ground like great drops of blood" (Luke 22:44). His close friends James and John, whom he had asked if they could drink the cup that he was going to drink, were there with him but fast asleep, unable to stay awake with him in his sorrow. In his immense loneliness, he fell on his face and cried out: "My Father, if it is possible, let this cup pass me by" (Matthew 26:39). Jesus couldn't face it. Too much pain to hold, too much suffering to embrace, too much agony to live through. He didn't feel he could drink that cup filled to the brim with sorrows.

Why then could he still say yes? I can't fully answer that question, except to say that beyond all the abandonment experienced in body and mind Jesus still had a spiritual bond with the one he called Abba. He possessed a trust beyond betrayal, a surrender beyond despair, a love beyond all fears. This intimacy beyond all human intimacies made it possible for Jesus to allow the request to let the cup pass him by become a prayer directed to the one who had called him "My Beloved." Notwithstanding his anguish, that bond of love had not been broken. It couldn't be felt in the body, nor thought through in the mind. But it was there, beyond all feelings and thoughts, and it maintained the communion underneath all disruptions. It was that spiritual sinew, that intimate communion with his Father, that made him hold on to the cup and pray: "My Father, let it be as you, not I, would have it" (Matthew 26:39).

Jesus didn't throw the cup away in despair. No, he kept it in his hands, willing to drink it to the dregs. This was not a show of willpower, staunch determination, or great heroism. This was a deep spiritual yes to Abba, the lover of his wounded heart.

When I contemplate my own sorrow-filled heart, when I think of my little community of people with mental handicaps and their assistants, when I see the poor of Toronto, and the immense anguish of men, women, and children far and wide on our planet, then I wonder where the great yes has to come from. In my own heart and the hearts of my fellow people, I hear the loud cry "O God, if it is possible, let this cup of sorrow pass us by." I hear it in the voice of the young man with AIDS begging for food on Yonge Street, in the little cries of starving children, in the screams of tortured prisoners, in the angry shouts of those who protest against nuclear proliferation and the destruction of the planet's ecological balance, and in the endless pleas for justice and peace all over the world. It is a prayer rising up to God not as incense but as a wild flame.

From where then will come that great yes? "Let it be as you, not I will have it." Who can say yes when the voice of love hasn't been heard! Who can say yes when there is no Abba to speak to? Who can say yes when there is no moment of consolation?

In the midst of Jesus' anguished prayer asking his Father to take his cup of sorrow away, there was one moment of consolation. Only the Evangelist Luke mentions it. He says: "Then an angel appeared to him, coming from heaven to give him strength" (Luke 22:43).

In the midst of the sorrows is consolation, in the midst of the darkness is light, in the midst of the despair is hope, in the midst of Babylon is a glimpse of Jerusalem, and in the midst of the army of demons is the consoling angel. The cup of sorrow, inconceivable as it seems, is also the cup of joy. Only when we discover this in our own life can we consider drinking it.

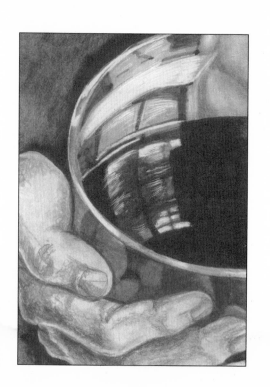

Chapter 3

THE CUP OF JOY

After my nine years at the Daybreak community, Adam, Michael, Bill, Tracy, Susanne, Loretta, David, Francis, Patrick, Janice, Carol, Gordie, George, and many others who live at the heart of our community have become my friends. More than friends, they are an intimate part of my daily life. Although they still are as handicapped as when I first met them, I seldom think of them as people with handicaps. I think of them as brothers and sisters with whom I share my life. I laugh with them, cry with them, eat dinners with them, go to the movies with them, pray and celebrate with them—in short, live my life with them. They truly fill me with immense joy.

After caring for Adam for a few months, I was no longer afraid of him. Waking him up in the morning, giving him a bath and brushing his teeth, shaving his beard and feeding him breakfast had created such a bond between us—a bond beyond words and visible signs of recognition—that I started to miss him when we couldn't be together. My time with him had become a time of prayer, silence, and quiet intimacy. Adam had become a true peacemaker for me, a man who loved and trusted me even when I made the water for his bath too hot or too cold, cut him with the razor, or gave him the wrong type of clothes to wear.

His epileptic seizures no longer scared me either. They simply caused me to slow down, forget about other obligations, and stay with him, covering him with heavy blankets to keep him warm. His difficult and very slow walk no longer irritated me but gave me an opportunity to stand behind him, put my arms around his waist, and speak encouraging words as he took one careful step after the other. His spilling a glass full of orange juice or dropping his spoon with food on the floor no longer made me panic but simply made me clean up. Knowing Adam became a privilege for me. Who can be as close to another human being as I could be to Adam? Who can spend a few hours each day with a man who gives you all his confidence and trust? Isn't that what joy is?

And Michael, Adam's brother: what a gift his friendship became! He became the only one in the community who calls me "Father Henri." Every time he says that, there is a smile on his face, suggesting that he really should be a Father too! With his halting, stuttering voice, he keeps saying, pointing to the large stole around my neck, "I . . . want . . . that . . . too . . . Father." When Michael is sad because his brother is sick, or because he has many seizures himself, or because someone he loves is leaving, he comes to me, puts his arms around me, and lets his tears flow freely. Then after a while he grabs me by the shoulder, looks at me, and with a big smile breaking through his tears he says: "You are . . . a . . . funny . . . Father!" When we pray together, he often points to his heart and says: "I feel . . . it. . . here . . . here in my heart." But as we hold hands, there is that immense joy that emerges from our shared sorrow.

Bill, the man with so many setbacks in his life, has become my special companion. He often comes with me on speaking trips. We have gone to Washington, New York, Los Angeles, and many other places over the years, and wherever we go, Bill's cheerful presence is as important as my many words. Bill loves to tell jokes. In his simple, direct, unselfconscious way, he entertains people for hours, whether they are wealthy or poor, dignitaries or simple folks, bishops or table servers, members of parliament or elevator operators. For Bill, everyone is important and everyone deserves to hear his jokes. But at moments Bill's sorrows can become too much for him. Sometimes when he talks about Adam, who cannot talk, or Tracy, who cannot walk, he bursts into tears. Then he puts his arms on my shoulders and cries openly, without embarrassment. And after a while his smile returns and he continues his story.

Then there is Tracy's radiant smile when a friend comes to see her, Loretta's gentle care for those who are much more handicapped than she, and the many little ways in which David, Janice, Carol, Gordie, George, and the others pay attention to each other and to their assistants. They all are true signs of joy.

It is not surprising that many young men and women from all over the world want to come to Daybreak to be close to these special people. Yes, they *come* to care for them and help them in their needs. But they *stay* because those they came to care for have brought them a joy and peace they had not been able to find anywhere else. Sure, the handicapped members of Daybreak put them in touch with their own handicaps, their own inner wounds and sorrows, but the joy that comes from living together in a fellowship of the weak makes the sorrow not just tolerable but a source of gratitude.

My own life in this community has been immensely joyful, even though I had never suffered so much, cried so much, and anguished so much as at Daybreak. Nowhere am I as well known as in this little community. It is totally impossible to hide my impatience, my anger, my frustration, and my depression from people who are so in touch with their own weakness. My needs for friendship, affection, and affirmation are right there for everyone to see. I have never experienced so deeply that the true nature of priesthood is a compassionate-being-with. Jesus' priesthood is described in the letter to the Hebrews as one of solidarity with human suffering. Calling myself a priest today radically challenges me to let go of every distance, every little pedestal, every ivory tower, and just to connect my own vulnerability with the vulnerability of those I live with. And what a joy that is! The joy of belonging, of being part of, of not being different.

Somehow my life at Daybreak has given me eyes to discover joy where many others see only sorrow. Talking with a homeless man on a Toronto street doesn't feel so frightening anymore. Soon money is not the main issue. It becomes: "Where are you from? Who are your friends? What is happening in your life?" Eyes meet, hands touch, and there is— yes, often completely unexpected—a smile, a burst of laughter, and a true moment of joy. The sorrow is still there, but something has changed by my no longer standing in front of others but sitting with them and sharing a moment of togetherness.

And the immense suffering of the world? How can there be joy among the dying, the hungry, the prostitutes, the refugees and the prisoners? How does anyone dare to speak about joy in the face of the unspeakable human sorrows surrounding us?

And yet, it is there! For anyone who has the courage to enter our human sorrows deeply, there is a revelation of joy, hidden like a precious stone in the wall of a dark cave. I got a glimpse of that while living with a very poor family in Pamplona Alta, one of the "young towns" at the outskirts of Lima, Peru. The poverty there was greater than any I had seen before, but when I think back on my three months with Pablo, Maria, and their children, my memories are filled with laughter, smiles, hugs, simple games, and long evenings just sitting around telling stories. Joy, real joy was there, not a joy based on success, progress, or the solution of their poverty, but bursting forth from the resilient human spirit, fully alive in the midst of all odds. And when Heather, the daughter of New York friends, recently returned from ten months' relief work in Rwanda, she had seen more than despair. She had also seen hope, courage, love, trust, and true care. Her heart was deeply troubled, but not crushed. She has been able to continue her life in the United States with a greater commitment to work for peace and justice. The joys of living were stronger than the sorrows of death.

The cup of life is the cup of joy as much as it is the cup of sorrow. It is the cup in which sorrows and joys, sadness and gladness, mourning and dancing are never separated. If joys could not be where sorrows are, the cup of life would never be drinkable. That is why we have to hold the cup in our hands and look carefully to see the joys hidden in our sorrows.

Can we look up to Jesus as to the man of joys? It seems impossible to see joy in the tortured, naked body hanging with outstretched arms on a wooden cross. Still, the cross of Jesus is often presented as a glorious throne on which the King is seated. There the body of Jesus is portrayed not as racked by flagellation and crucifixion but as a beautiful, luminous body with sacred wounds.

The cross of San Damiano that spoke to St. Francis of Assisi is a good example. It shows the crucified Jesus as a victorious Jesus. The cross is surrounded by splendid gold; the body of Jesus is a perfect, immaculate human body; the horizontal beam on which he hangs is painted as the open grave from which Jesus rose; and all those gathered under the cross with Mary and John are full of joy. At the top we can see God's hand, surrounded by angels, drawing Jesus back into heaven.

This is a resurrection cross, in which we see Jesus lifted up in glory. Jesus' words "When I am lifted up from the earth, I shall draw all people to myself" (John 12:32) refer not only to his crucifixion but also to his resurrection. Being lifted up means not only being lifted up as the crucified one but also being lifted up as the risen one. It speaks not only about agony but also about ecstasy, not only about sorrow but also about joy.

Jesus makes this very clear when he says: "As Moses lifted up the snake in the desert, so must the Son of man be lifted up, so that everyone who believes may have eternal life in him" (John 3:13-14). What Moses raised in the desert as a standard was a bronze serpent, healing everyone bitten by snakes who looked up at it (Numbers 21:8-9). The cross of Jesus is likewise the standard of healing, not just healing from physical wounds, but healing from the human condition of mortality. The risen Lord draws all people with him into his new and eternal life. Jesus who cries out, "My God, my God, why have you forsaken me?" (Matthew 27:47) also says in total surrender: "Father, into your hands I commit my spirit" (Luke 23:46). Jesus, who participated fully in all our pain, wants us to participate fully in his joy. Jesus the man of joy wants us to be the people of joy.

"Can you drink the cup that I am going to drink?" When Jesus brought this question to John and James, and when they impulsively answered with a big "We can," he made this terrifying, yet hope-filled prediction: "Very well; you shall drink my cup." The cup of Jesus would be their cup. What Jesus would live, they would live. Jesus didn't want his friends to suffer, but he knew that for them, as for him, suffering was the only and necessary way to glory. Later he would say to two of his disciples: "Was it not necessary that the Christ should suffer before entering into his glory?" (Luke 24:26). The "cup of sorrows" and the "cup of joys" cannot be separated. Jesus knew this, even though in the midst of his anguish in the garden, when his soul was "sorrowful to the point of death" (Matthew 26:38), he needed an angel from heaven to remind him of it. Our cup is often so full of pain that joy seems completely unreachable. When we are crushed like grapes, we cannot think of the wine we will become. The sorrow overwhelms us, makes us throw ourselves on the ground, face down, and sweat drops of blood. Then we need to be reminded that our cup of sorrow is also our cup of joy and that one day we will be able to taste the joy as fully as we now taste the sorrow.

Soon after the angel had given him strength, Jesus stood up and faced Judas and the cohort who had come to arrest him. When Peter drew his sword and struck the high priest's servant, Jesus said to him, "Put your sword back in its scabbard; am I not to drink the cup that the Father has given me?" (John 18:10-11).

Now Jesus is no longer overcome by anguish. He stands in front of his enemies with great dignity and inner freedom. He holds his cup filled with sorrow but with joy too. It is the joy of knowing that what he is about to undergo is the will of his

Father and will lead him to the fulfillment of his mission. The Evangelist John shows us the enormous power that emanates from Jesus. He writes: "Knowing everything that was to happen to him, Jesus came forward and said [to Judas and the cohort]: 'Who are you looking for?' They answered, 'Jesus the Nazarene.' He said, 'I am he.' . . . When Jesus said to them, 'I am he,' they moved back and fell on the ground" (John 18:4-6).

Jesus' unconditional yes to his Father had empowered him to drink his cup, not in passive resignation but with the full knowledge that the hour of his death would also be the hour of his glory. His yes made his surrender a creative act, an act that could bear much fruit. His yes took away the fatality of the interruption of his ministry. Instead of a final irrevocable end, his death became the beginning of a new life. Indeed, his yes enabled him to trust fully in the rich harvest the dying grain would yield.

Joys are hidden in sorrows! I know this from my own times of depression. I know it from living with people with mental handicaps. I know it from looking into the eyes of patients, and from being with the poorest of the poor. We keep forgetting this truth and become overwhelmed by our own darkness. We easily lose sight of our joys and speak of our sorrows as the only reality there is.

We need to remind each other that the cup of sorrow is also the cup of joy, that precisely what causes us sadness can become the fertile ground for gladness. Indeed, we need to be angels for each other, to give each other strength and consolation. Because only when we fully realize that the cup of life is not only a cup of sorrow but also a cup of joy will we be able to drink it.

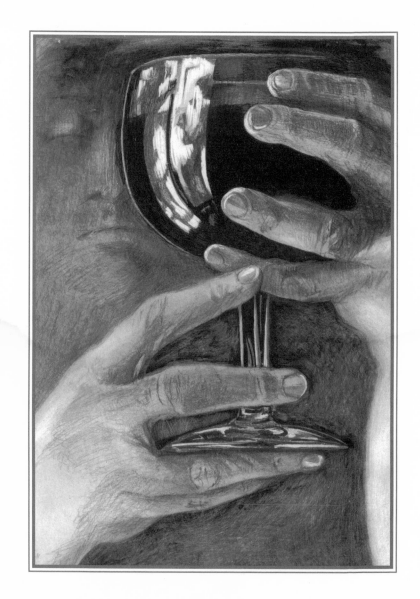

Part 2

LIFTING
THE CUP

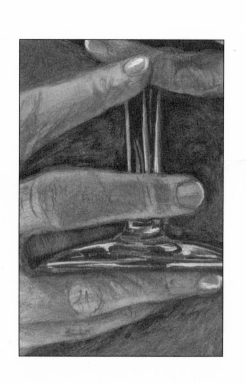

Chapter 4

LIFTING

Good manners were very important in our family, especially table manners.

In the hall of our home hung a large bell. Ten minutes before dinner, my father rang the bell loudly and announced: "Dinnertime, everybody wash their hands."

There were many "table sins": elbows on the table, heaping up food on your spoon or fork, eating fast, making noises, chewing with your mouth open, not using your fork and knife while eating meat, using your knife to cut spaghetti. Many of our meals were interspersed with my father's little commands: "Elbows off the table," "Wait until everyone is served," and "Don't talk as you eat."

As I became older, I was allowed to have a glass of wine. It was a sign of adulthood. In 1950, when I was eighteen years old, drinking wine was a luxury. In France and Italy, wine at dinner was part of daily life, but in Holland it was a sign of a festive occasion. When we had wine there were special rituals: tasting and approving the wine, saying a few good words about it, pouring it into the glasses—only half full—and, most important of all, lifting it for a toast.

No one in our family would ever drink from his or her glass before everyone had been served and my father had lifted up his glass, looked at each of us, spoken a word of welcome, and emphasized the uniqueness of the occasion. Then, with his glass he touched my mother's glass and the glasses of his guests and drank a little. It always was a solemn and important moment, a moment with a sacred quality. In later years, when wine was no longer so special, when glasses were filled to the brim, and when people drank without lifting their glasses or offering a toast, I always felt that something was missing, yes, even that something was lost.

Lifting up the cup is an invitation to affirm and celebrate life together. As we lift up the cup of life and look each other in the eye, we say: "Let's not be anxious or afraid. Let's hold our cup together and greet each other. Let us not hesitate to acknowledge the reality of our lives and encourage each other to be grateful for the gifts we have received."

We say to each other: in Latin, *"Prosit"* (be well); in German, *"Zum Wohl"* (to your well-being); in Dutch, *"Op je gezondheid"* (to your health); in English, "Cheers"; in French, *"A votre santé"* (to your health); in Italian, *"Alla tua salute"* (to your health); in Polish, *"Sto lat"* (a hundred years); in Ukrainian, *"Na zdorvia"* (to your health); in Hebrew, *"L'chaim"* (to life).

The best summary of all these wishes is, "to life." We lift the cup to life, to affirm our life together and celebrate it as a gift from God. When each of us can hold firm our own cup, with its many sorrows and joys, claiming it as our unique life, then too, can we lift it up for others to see and encourage them to lift up their lives as well. Thus, as we lift up our cup in a fearless gesture, proclaiming that we will support each other in our common journey, we create community.

Nothing is sweet or easy about community. Community is a fellowship of people who do not hide their joys and sorrows but make them visible to each other in a gesture of hope. In community we say: "Life is full of gains and losses, joys and sorrows, ups and downs—but we do not have to live it alone. We want to drink our cup together and thus celebrate the truth that the wounds of our individual lives, which seem intolerable when lived alone, become sources of healing when we live them as part of a fellowship of mutual care."

Community is like a large mosaic. Each little piece seems so insignificant. One piece is bright red, another cold blue or dull green, another warm purple, another sharp yellow, another shining gold. Some look precious, others ordinary. Some look valuable, others worthless. Some look gaudy, others delicate. As individual stones, we can do little with them except compare them and judge their beauty and value. When, however, all these little stones are brought together in one big mosaic portraying the face of Christ, who would ever question the importance of any one of them? If one of them, even the least spectacular one, is missing, the face is incomplete. Together in the one mosaic, each little stone is indispensable and makes a unique contribution to the glory of God. That's community, a fellowship of little people who together make God visible in the world.

Lifting our lives to others happens every time we speak or act in ways that make our lives lives for others. When we are fully able to embrace our own lives, we discover that what we claim we also want to proclaim. A life well held is indeed a life for others. We stop wondering whether our life is better or worse than others and start seeing clearly that when we live our life for others we not only claim our individuality but also proclaim our unique place in the mosaic of the human family.

So often we are inclined to keep our lives hidden. Shame and guilt prevent us from letting others know what we are living. We think: "If my family and friends knew the dark cravings of my heart and my strange mental wanderings, they would push me away and exclude me from their company." But the opposite is true. When we dare to lift our cup and let our friends know what is in it, they will be encouraged to lift their cups and share with us their own anxiously hidden secrets. The greatest healing often takes place when we no longer feel isolated by our shame and guilt and discover that others often feel what we feel and think what we think and have the fears, apprehensions, and preoccupations we have.

Lifting our cup means sharing our life so we can celebrate it. When we truly believe we are called to lay down our lives for our friends, we must dare to take the risk to let others know what we are living. The important question is, "Do we have a circle of trustworthy friends where we feel safe enough to be intimately known and called to an always greater maturity?" Just as we lift up our glasses to people we trust and love, so we lift up the cup of our life to those from whom we do not want to have secrets and with whom we want to form community.

When we do want to drink our cup and drink it to the bottom, we need others who are willing to drink their cups with us. We need community, a community in which confession and celebration are always present together. We have to be willing to let others know us if we want them to celebrate life with us. When we lift our cups and say "to life," we should be talking about real lives, not only hard, painful, sorrowful lives, but also lives so full of joy that celebration becomes a spontaneous response.

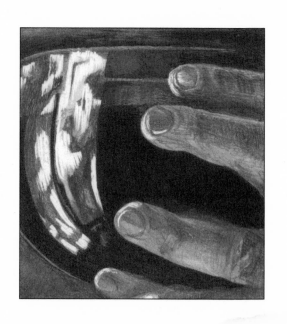

Chapter 5

THE CUP OF BLESSINGS

Lifting the cup is offering a blessing. The cup of sorrow and joy, when lifted for others "to life," becomes the cup of blessings.

I have a very lively memory connected with the cup of sorrow and joy becoming the cup of blessings. A few years ago, one of the handicapped members of the Daybreak community had to spend a few months in a mental hospital near Toronto for psychological evaluation. His name is Trevor. Trevor and I had become close friends over the years. He loved me and I loved him. Whenever he saw me coming, he ran up to me with a great radiant smile. Often he went into the fields and collected wildflowers for me. He always wanted to assist me in the celebrations of the Eucharist and had a fine sense for ceremony and ritual.

During the time Trevor was away from Daybreak, I decided to go see him. I called the hospital chaplain and asked him if I could visit my friend. He said I was welcome to come and wondered if it would be all right if he invited some of the ministers and priests in the area and some members of the hospital staff to have lunch with me. Without thinking much about the implications of this request, I said immediately, "Sure, that will be fine."

When I arrived at 11:00 A.M., a large group of clergy and hospital personnel was waiting for me, and they welcomed me warmly. I looked around for Trevor, but he wasn't there. So I said: "I came here to visit Trevor. Can you tell me where I can find him?" The hospital chaplain said: "You can be with him after lunch." I was stunned and said, "But didn't you invite him for lunch?" "No, no," he said, "that's impossible. Staff and patients cannot have lunch together. Moreover, we have reserved the Golden Room for this occasion, and no patient has ever been allowed in that room. It is for staff only." "Well," I said, "I will only have lunch with you all when Trevor can be there too. Trevor and I are close friends. It is for him that I came, and I am sure he would love to join us for lunch." I noticed some mixed reactions to my words, but after some whispering I was told that I could bring Trevor with me to the Golden Room.

I found Trevor on the hospital grounds, as always, looking for flowers. When he saw me his face lit up, and he ran up to me as if we had never been apart and said: "Henri, here are some flowers for you." Together we went to the Golden Room. The table was beautifully set, and about twenty-five people had gathered around it. Trevor and I were the last to sit down.

After the opening prayer, Trevor walked to the side table where there were different drinks: wine, soft drinks, and juices. He said: "Henri, I want a Coke." I poured him a Coke, took a glass of wine for myself, and returned to the table.

People were making small talk. Many of the guests were strangers trying to get to know each other. The general atmosphere was quiet, somewhat solemn. I got quickly involved in a conversation with my right-hand neighbor and didn't pay much attention to Trevor. But suddenly Trevor stood up, took his glass of Coke, lifted it, and said with a loud voice and a big smile: "Ladies and gentlemen . . . a toast!" Everyone dropped their conversation and turned to Trevor with puzzled and somewhat anxious faces. I could read their thoughts: "What in the heck is this patient going to do? Better be careful."

But Trevor had no worries. He looked at everybody and said: "Lift up your glasses." Everyone obeyed. And then, as if it were the most obvious thing to do, he started to sing: "When you're happy and you know it . . . lift your glass. When you're happy and you know it . . . lift your glass. When you're happy and you know it, when you're happy and you know it, when you're happy and you know it . . . lift your glass." As he sang, people's faces relaxed and started to smile. Soon a few joined Trevor in his song, and not long after everyone was standing, singing loudly under Trevor's direction.

Trevor's toast radically changed the mood in the Golden Room. He had brought these strangers together and made them feel at home. His beautiful smile and his fearless joy had broken down the barriers between staff and patients and created a happy family of caring people. With his unique blessing, Trevor had set the tone for a joyful and fruitful meeting. The cup of sorrow and joy had become the cup of blessings.

Many people feel cursed—cursed by God with illnesses, losses, handicaps, and misfortunes. They believe their cup doesn't carry any blessings. It is the cup of God's wrath, the cup Jeremiah speaks of when he says:

> For Yahweh, the God of Israel said this to me, "Take this cup of the wine of wrath and make all the nations to whom I send you drink it; they will drink and reel and lose their wits, because of the sword I am sending among them. . . . You will say to them, 'Yahweh Sabaoth, the God of Israel, says this: Drink! Get drunk! Vomit! Fall, never to rise again, before the sword that I am sending among you!' If they refuse to take the cup from your hand and drink, you will say to them, 'Yahweh Sabaoth says this: You must drink! Look, for a start, I am bringing disaster on the city that bears my name, so are you likely to go unpunished? You certainly will not go unpunished, for next I shall summon a sword against all the inhabitants of the land, Yahweh declares' " (Jeremiah 25:15-16, 27-29).

This is not a cup to lift "to life." It only brings misery. It is not surprising that no one wants to get close to the vengeful god that Jeremiah depicts. No blessing is found there. But when Jesus takes the cup on the evening before his death, it is not the cup of wrath but the cup of blessings. It is the cup of a new and everlasting covenant, the cup that unites us with God and with one another in a community of love. Paul writes to the people of Corinth: "I am talking to you as sensible people; weigh up for yourselves what I have to say. The blessing-cup, which we bless, is it not a sharing in the blood of Christ?" (1 Corinthians 10:15-16).

The immense suffering of humanity can easily be understood as a sign of God's wrath, as a punishment. It often was understood that way, and it often still is. The Psalmist says: "Yahweh is holding a cup filled with a heady blend of wine; he will pour it, they will drink it to the dregs, all the wicked on earth will drink it" (Psalm 75:8). And we, looking at the horrors that plague our world, are saying, "How can there be a loving God when all this is happening? It must be a cruel, spiteful God who allows human beings to suffer so much!"

Jesus, however, took upon himself all this suffering and lifted it up on the cross, not as a curse but as a blessing. Jesus made the cup of God's wrath into a cup of blessings. That's the mystery of the Eucharist. Jesus died for us so that we may live. He poured out his blood for us so that we may find new life. He gave himself away for us, so that we can live in community. He became for us food and drink so that we can be fed for everlasting life. That is what Jesus meant when he took the cup and said: "This cup is the new covenant in my blood poured out for you" (Luke 22:20). The Eucharist is that sacred mystery through which what we lived as a curse, we now live as a blessing. Our suffering can no longer be a divine punishment. Jesus transformed it as the way to new life. His blood, and ours too, now can become martyr's blood — blood that witnesses to a new covenant, a new communion, a new community.

When we lift the cup of our life and share with one another our sufferings and joys in mutual vulnerability, the new covenant can become visible among us. The surprise of it all is that it is often the least among us who reveal to us that our cup is a cup of blessings.

Trevor did what nobody else could have done. He transformed a group of strangers into a community of love by his simple, unself-conscious blessing. He, a meek man, became the living Christ among us. The cup of blessings is the cup the meek have to offer to us.

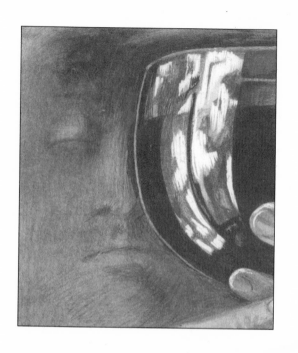

Chapter 6

TO LIFE

We lift the cups of our lives to bring life to each other.

In the Daybreak community, celebration is an essential part of our life together. We celebrate birthdays and anniversaries, we celebrate those who arrive and those who depart, we celebrate birth and death, we celebrate commitments made and commitments renewed.

In our community there are many parties. Parties are usually happy events, during which we eat and drink, sing and dance, give speeches, talk and laugh a lot. But a celebration is something more than just than a party. A celebration is an occasion to lift up each other's lives—whether in a joyful or a sorrowful moment—and deepen our bonds with each other.

To celebrate life is to raise up life, make it visible to each other, affirm it in its concreteness, and be grateful for it.

One very moving celebration I remember was that of Bill's *Life Story Book*. A *Life Story Book* is a collection of photographs, stories, and letters put together as a sort of biography. When Bill came to Daybreak as a sixteen-year-old, he brought few memories with him. He had had a very troublesome childhood and hardly any consistent experiences of love and friendship. His past was so broken, so painful, and so lonely that he had chosen to forget it. He was a man without a history.

But during twenty-five years at Daybreak, he gradually has become a different person. He has made friends. He has developed a close relationship with a family he can visit on weekends or holidays, joined a bowling club, learned woodworking, and traveled with me to places far and wide. Over the years he has created a life worth remembering. He even found the freedom and the courage to recall some of his painful childhood experiences and to reclaim his deceased parents as people who had given him life and love notwithstanding their limitations.

Now there was enough material for a *Life Story Book* because now there was a beautiful although painful story to tell. Many friends wrote letters to Bill telling him what they remembered about him. Others sent photographs or newspaper clippings about events he had been part of, and others just made drawings that expressed their love for him. After six months of work, the book was finally ready, and it was time to celebrate, not just the new book but Bill's life, which it symbolized.

Many came together for the occasion in the Dayspring Chapel. Bill held the book and lifted it up for all to see. It was a beautifully colored ring binder with many artistically decorated pages. Although it was Bill's book, it was the work of many people.

Then we blessed the book and Bill, who held it. I prayed that this book might help Bill let many people know what a beautiful man he is and what a good life he was living. I also prayed that Bill would remember all the moments of his life—his joys as well as his sorrows—with a grateful heart.

While I prayed tears started to flow from Bill's eyes. When I finished he threw his arms around me and cried loudly. His tears fell on my shoulder while everyone in the circle looked at us with a deep understanding of what was happening. Bill's life had been lifted up for all to see, and he had been able to say it was a life to be grateful for.

Now Bill takes his *Life Story Book* with him on his trips. He shows it to people as a man who believes his life is not something to be ashamed of. To the contrary, it is a gift for others.

The cup of sorrow and joy, when lifted for others to see and celebrate, becomes a cup to life. It is so easy for us to live truncated lives because of hard things that have happened in our past, which we prefer not to remember. Often the burdens of our past seem too heavy for us to carry alone. Shame and guilt make us hide part of ourselves and thus make us live half lives.

We truly need each other to claim all of our lives and to live them to the fullest. We need each other to move beyond our guilt and shame and to become grateful, not just for our successes and accomplishments but also for our failures and shortcomings. We need to be able to let our tears flow freely, tears of sorrow as well as tears of joy, tears that are as rain on dry ground. As we thus lift our lives for each other, we can truly say: "To life," because all we have lived now becomes the fertile soil for the future.

But lifting our cup to life is much more than saying good things about each other. It is much more than offering good wishes. It means that we take all we have ever lived and bring it to the present moment as a gift for others, a gift to celebrate.

Mostly we are willing to look back at our lives and say: "I am grateful for the *good* things that brought me to this place."

But when we lift our cup to life, we must dare to say: "I am grateful for *all* that has happened to me and led me to this moment." This gratitude which embraces all of our past is what makes our life a true gift for others, because this gratitude erases bitterness, resentments, regret, and revenge as well as all jealousies and rivalries. It transforms our past into a fruitful gift for the future, and makes our life, all of it, into a life that gives life.

The enormous individualism of our society, in which so much emphasis is on "doing it yourself," prevents us from lifting our lives for each other. But each time we dare to step beyond our fear, to be vulnerable and lift our cup, our own and other people's lives will blossom in unexpected ways.

Then we too will find the strength to drink our cup and drink it to the bottom.

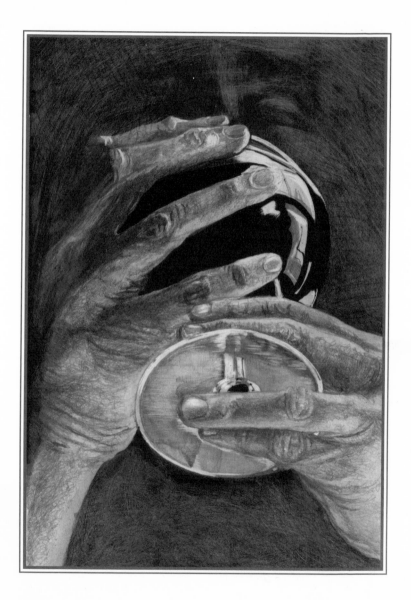

Part 3

DRINKING
THE CUP

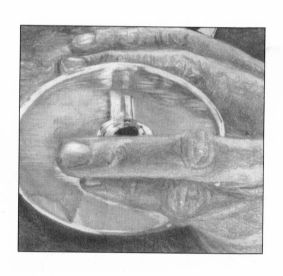

Chapter 7

DRINKING

The cup that we hold and lift we must drink.

I have very vivid memories of my first year at the University of Nijmegen in Holland. I had just been ordained a priest, and Cardinal Alfrink had sent me to the Catholic university to work for a degree in psychology. But before the school year started, I had to undergo a long hazing process to be accepted into the student society and to become a member of a fraternity. Drinking beer was definitely one of the ways to get in! I wasn't used to drinking that much beer and had a hard time showing any prowess in this domain. But once I was finally admitted into the society and had made some friends in the fraternity, "having a drink together" became an expression for sharing, personal attention, good conversation, and the deepening of fellowship. "Let's have a beer!" "Can you join me for coffee?" "Let's meet for tea." "May I offer you a Heineken?"

"What about another glass of wine?" "Come on, don't be shy, let me pour you another . . . you deserve it!" These and other similar ways of speaking created an atmosphere of companionship and conviviality.

In whatever country or culture we find ourselves, having a drink together is a sign of friendship, intimacy, and peace. Being thirsty is often not the main reason to drink. We drink to "break the ice," to enter into a conversation, to show good intention, to express friendship and goodwill, to set the stage for a romantic moment, to be open, vulnerable, accessible. It is no surprise that people who are angry at us, or who come to accuse us or harass us, won't accept a drink from us. They would rather say: "I will come straight to the point of my being here." Refusing a drink is avoiding intimacy.

At worst, drinking together is saying, "We trust each other enough that we don't want to poison each other." At best, it is saying, "I want to get close to you and celebrate life with you." It breaks through the boundaries that separate us and invites us to recognize our shared humanity. Thus, drinking together can be a true spiritual event, affirming our unity as children of one God.

The world is full of places to drink: bars, pubs, coffee and tea rooms. Even when we go out to eat, the waiter's first question is always "Can I offer you something to drink?" That is also one of the first questions we ask our guests when they enter our home.

It seems that most of our drinking takes place in a context in which we feel, at least for a moment, at home with ourselves and safe with others. Drinking a cup of coffee to interrupt work for a moment, stopping for tea in the afternoon, having a "quick drink" before dinner, taking a glass of wine before going to bed—all these are moments to say to ourselves or others: "It is good to be alive in the midst of all that is going on, and I want to be reminded of that."

Drinking the cup of life makes our own everything we are living. It is saying, "This is my life," but also "I want this to be my life." Drinking the cup of life is fully appropriating and internalizing our own unique existence, with all its sorrows and joys.

It is not easy to do this. For a long time we might not feel capable of accepting our own life; we might keep fighting for a better or at least a different life. Often a deep protest against our "fate" rises in us. We didn't choose our country, our parents, the color of our skin, our sexual orientation. We didn't even choose our character, intelligence, physical appearance, or mannerisms. Sometimes we want to do every possible thing to change the circumstances of our life. We wish we were in another body, lived in another time, or had another mind! A cry can come out of our depths: "Why do I have to be this person? I didn't ask for it, and I don't want it."

But as we gradually come to befriend our own reality, to look with compassion at our own sorrows and joys, and as we are able to discover the unique potential of our way of being in the world, we can move beyond our protest, put the cup of our life to our lips and drink it, slowly, carefully, but fully.

Often when we wish to comfort people, we say: "Well, it is sad this has happened to you, but try to make the best of it." But "making the best of it" is not what drinking the cup is about. Drinking our cup is not simply adapting ourselves to a bad situation and trying to use it as well as we can. Drinking our cup is a hopeful, courageous, and self-confident way of living. It is standing in the world with head erect, solidly rooted in the knowledge of who we are, facing the reality that surrounds us and responding to it from our hearts.

The great figures in history looked deeply into their cups and drank from them without fear. Whether they were famous or not, they knew that the life which was given to them was given to live to its fullness in the presence of God and God's people, and thus bear much fruit. They needed to make it bear fruit. Jesus, the carpenter's son from Nazareth—"Can anything good come from Nazareth?" people asked

(John 1:46)—drank his cup to the bitter end. All his disciples did too, different as they may have been.

Spiritual greatness has nothing to do with being greater than others. It has everything to do with being as great as each of us can be. True sanctity is precisely drinking our own cup and trusting that by thus fully claiming our own, irreplaceable journey, we can become a source of hope for many. Vincent van Gogh, miserable and brokenhearted as he was, believed without question in his vocation to paint, and he went as far as he could with what little he had. This is true for Francis of Assisi, Dorothy Day of New York, and Oscar Romero of San Salvador. Small people, but great in drinking their cups to the full.

How then can we, in the midst of our ordinary daily lives, drink our cup, the cup of sorrow and the cup of joy? How can we fully appropriate what is given to us? Somehow we know that when we do not drink our cup and thus avoid the sorrow as well as the joy of living, our lives become inauthentic, insincere, superficial, and boring. We become puppets moved up and down, left and right by the puppeteers of this world. We become objects, yes, victims of other people's interests and desires. But we don't have to be victims. We can choose to drink the cup of our life with the deep conviction that by drinking it we will find our true freedom. Thus, we will discover that the cup of sorrow and joy we are drinking is the cup of salvation.

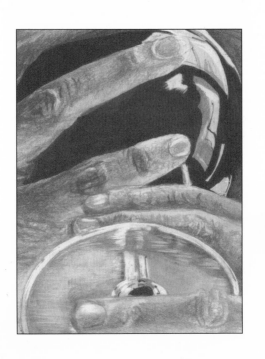

Chapter 8

THE CUP OF SALVATION

Gordie Henry, who has Down's syndrome, is one of the core members of the Daybreak community. Once he said to me, "What is good about our life is that you make so many friends. What is hard about our life is that so many friends leave." With this simple observation Gordie touched the place where joy and sorrow are embracing each other. As a longtime member of Daybreak, Gordie has had many assistants come to live with him. They came from various countries, sometimes for a summer, sometimes for a year, sometimes for many years. They all loved Gordie very much, and Gordie came to love them. Strong attachments and deep bonds of friendship developed.

But sooner or later, the assistants had to leave. Some got married, some returned to school, some lost their work permits, some looked for a new direction in life, and some discovered that community life wasn't for them. Gordie, however, stayed, and felt the intense pain of the many separations.

One day, Jean Vanier, the founder of l'Arche, came to visit Daybreak. He gathered the whole community around him and said, "What questions would you most like to ask me?" Thelus, one of the core members who had lived at Daybreak as long as Gordie, raised her hand and said: "Why are people leaving all the time?" Jean understood this question was not just Thelus' question but also Gordie's question and the question of all long-term Daybreak members.

He gently moved closer to her and said: "You know, Thelus, that *is* the most important question you can ask. Because you and many others want to make Daybreak your home, where you can feel well loved and well protected. What then does it mean when so often someone you love, and who loves you, leaves your home, sometimes for good? Why then do you have to suffer the pain of so many departures? It may feel as if people do not really love you! Because if they love you, why would they leave you?"

As he was speaking, everyone looked at him very attentively. They knew this man truly understood their pain and sincerely cared for them. They wanted to hear what he had to say. With great gentleness and compassion, Jean looked at everyone who was listening and said: "You know, your joy and your pain give you a mission.

Those who came to live with you, from whom you received much and to whom you gave much, aren't just leaving you. You are sending them back to their schools, their homes, and their families, to bring some of the love they have lived with you. It's hard. It's painful to let them go. But when you realize that this is a mission, you will be able to send your friends to continue their journeys without losing the joy they brought you."

These simple words entered deep into our hearts because they made us look differently at what had seemed such a harsh tearing apart. The cup of joy and sorrow had become the cup of salvation.

Drinking the cup of sorrow and joy is only possible when it bring us health, strength, freedom, hope, courage—new life. Nobody will drink the cup of life when it makes us sick and miserable. We can only drink it when it is a cup of salvation.

This is beautifully expressed in Psalm 116:
The Lord is merciful and upright,
our God is tenderness. . . .
My trust does not fail even when I say,
"I am completely wretched."
In my terror I said,
"No human being can be relied on."
What return can I make to the Lord
for his generosity to me?
I shall take up the cup of salvation and call on the
name of the Lord.

(Psalm 116:5, 10-13, *New Jerusalem Bible.*
The word "Yahweh" is replaced by "Lord.")

Here the mystery of drinking the cup becomes clear. The coming and leaving of friends, the experiences of love and betrayal, of care and indifference, of generosity and stinginess can become the way to true human freedom. Yes, people who love us also disappoint us, moments of great satisfaction also reveal unfulfilled needs, being home also shows us our homelessness. But all of these tensions can create in us that deep, deep yearning for full freedom that is beyond any of the structures of our world.

Indeed, there is a mission emerging out of a life that is never pure sorrow or pure joy, a mission that makes us move far beyond our human limitations and reach out to total freedom, complete redemption, ultimate salvation.

Jesus drank the cup of his life. He experienced praise, adulation, admiration, and immense popularity. He also experienced rejection, ridicule, and mass hatred. At one moment people shouted "Hosanna"; a moment later they cried: "Crucify him." Jesus took it all in, not as a hero adored and then vilified, but as the one who had come to fulfill a mission and who kept his focus on that mission whatever the responses were. Jesus knew deep within himself that he had to drink the cup to accomplish the work his Abba—his dear Father—had given him. He knew that drinking the cup would bring him freedom, glory, and wholeness. He knew that drinking the cup would lead him beyond the entrapment of this world to complete liberation, beyond the agony of death to the splendor of the resurrection. This knowing had little to do with understanding or comprehending. It was a knowledge of a heart shaped in the garden of eternal love.

Thus the cup which Jesus was willing to drink, and which he drank until it was completely empty, became the cup of salvation. In the garden of Gethsemane, the garden of fear, Jesus' heart cried out with the psalmist: "No human being can be relied on. . . . I shall take up the cup of salvation and call on the name of the Lord." Drinking the cup of salvation means emptying the cup of sorrow and joy so that God can fill it with pure life.

"Salvation" is about being saved. But from what do we need to be saved? The traditional answer—and the good one—is sin and death. We are entrapped by sin and death as in a hunter's snare.

When we think for a moment of various addictions—alcohol, drug, food, gambling, sex—we get some idea of that entrapment.

In addition there are our many compulsions. We can feel compelled to act, speak, and even think in one way without being able to choose any other way. When people say: "Be sure you clean the room before you leave it, otherwise he gets raving mad!" or "Whatever she does, she first needs to wash her hands," we know that we are dealing with compulsive people.

Finally, all of us have our obsessions. An idea, a plan, a hobby can obsess us to such a degree that we become its slave.

These addictions, compulsions, and obsessions reveal our entrapments. They show our sinfulness because they take away our freedom as children of God and thus enslave us in a cramped, shrunken world. Sin makes us want to create our own lives according to our desires and wishes, ignoring the cup that is given to us. Sin makes us self-indulgent. St. Paul says: "When self-indulgence is at work the results are obvious: sexual vice, impurity, and sensuality, the worship of false gods and sorcery; antagonisms and rivalry, jealousy, bad temper and quarrels, disagreements, factions and malice, drunkenness, orgies and all such things" (Galatians 5:18-21).

Death too entraps us. Death is surrounding us on all sides: the threat of nuclear death; the reality of death caused by the many international, national, and ethnic conflicts; the death resulting from starvation and neglect; the death through abortion and euthanasia; and the death coming from the countless diseases that plague humanity, especially AIDS and cancer. Sooner or later the inevitability of our own deaths will catch up with us. In whatever direction we run, death is there, never leaving us completely alone. Not a day passes in which we are

O Holy Wisdom
in the stillness, with Mary,
we contemplate your presence
revealed to us
in word and sacrament,
in all creation.
We celebrate our call
to be a living praise to your glory
as we join all creation in proclaiming
your love to the ends of the earth.

October 1996 ~ October 1997

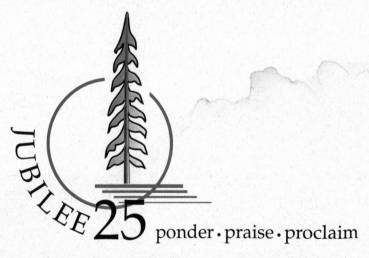

JUBILEE **25** ponder • praise • proclaim

Mary's Solitude • Saint Mary's • Notre Dame, IN 46556

not worried about the health of a family member, a friend, or ourselves. Not a day passes that we aren't reminded of those snares of death.

Sin and death entrap us. Drinking the cup, as Jesus did, is the way out of that trap. It is the way to salvation. It is a hard way, a painful way, a way we want to avoid at all costs. Often it even seems an impossible way. Still, unless we are willing to drink our cup, real freedom will elude us. This is not only the freedom that comes after we have completely emptied our cup—that is, after we have died. No, this freedom comes to us every time we drink from the cup of life, whether a little or much.

Salvation is not only a goal for the afterlife. Salvation is a reality of every day that we can taste here and now. When I sit down with Adam and help him eat, chat with Bill about our next trip, have coffee with Susanne and breakfast with David, when I embrace Michael, kiss Patsy, or pray with Gordie, salvation is right there. And when we sit together around the low altar table and I offer to all present the glass cup filled with wine, I can announce with great certainty: "This is the cup of salvation."

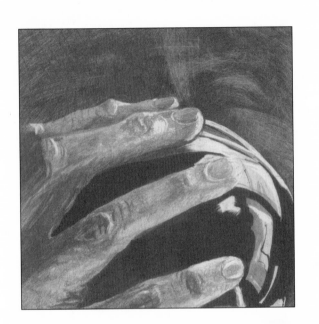

Chapter 9

To the Bottom

The question now is: How do we drink the cup of salvation?

We have to drink our cup slowly, tasting every mouthful—all the way to the bottom! Living a complete life is drinking our cup until it is empty, trusting that God will fill it with everlasting life.

It is important, however, to be very specific when we deal with the question "How do we drink our cup?" We need some very concrete disciplines to help us fully appropriate and internalize our joys and sorrows and find in them our unique way to spiritual freedom. I would like to explore how three disciplines—the discipline of silence, the discipline of the word, and the discipline of action—can help us drink our cup of salvation.

The first way to drink our cup is in silence.

This might come as a surprise, since being silent seems like doing nothing, but it is precisely in silence that we confront our true selves. The sorrows of our lives often overwhelm us to such a degree that we will do everything not to face them. Radio, television, newspapers, books, films, but also hard work and a busy social life all can be ways to run away from ourselves and turn life into a long entertainment.

The word *entertainment* is important here. It means literally "to keep (*tain* from the Latin *tenere*) someone in between (*enter*)." Entertainment is everything that gets and keeps our mind away from things that are hard to face. Entertainment keeps us distracted, excited, or in suspense. Entertainment is often good for us. It gives us an evening or a day off from our worries and fears. But when we start living life as entertainment, we lose touch with our souls and become little more than spectators in a lifelong show. Even very useful and relevant work can become a way of forgetting who we really are. It is no surprise that for many people retirement is a fearful prospect. Who are we when there is nothing to keep us busy?

Silence is the discipline that helps us to go beyond the entertainment quality of our lives. There we can let our sorrows and joys emerge from their hidden place and look us in the face, saying: "Don't be afraid; you can look at your own journey, its dark and light sides, and discover your way to freedom." We may find silence in nature, in our own houses, in a church or meditation hall. But wherever we find it, we should cherish it. Because it is in silence that we can truly acknowledge who we are and gradually claim ourselves as a gift from God.

At first silence might only frighten us. In silence we start hearing the voices of darkness: our jealousy and anger, our resentment and desire for revenge, our lust and greed, and our pain over losses, abuses, and rejections. These voices are often noisy and boisterous. They may even deafen us. Our most spontaneous reaction is to run away from them and return to our entertainment.

But if we have the discipline to stay put and not let these dark voices intimidate us, they will gradually lose their strength and recede into the background, creating space for the softer, gentler voices of the light.

These voices speak of peace, kindness, gentleness, goodness, joy, hope, forgiveness, and, most of all, love. They might at first seem small and insignificant, and we may have a hard time trusting them. However, they are very persistent and they will grow stronger if we keep listening. They come from a very deep place and from very far. They have been speaking to us since before we were born, and they reveal to us that there is no darkness in the One who sent us into the world, only light.

They are part of God's voice calling us from all eternity: "My beloved child, my favorite one, my joy."

The enormous powers of our world keep drowning out these gentle voices. Still, they are the voices of truth. They are like the voice that Elijah heard on Mount Horeb. There God passed him not in a hurricane, an earthquake, or a fire but in "a light murmuring sound" (1 Kings 19:11-13). This sound takes away our fear and makes us realize that we can face reality, especially our own reality. Being in silence is the first way we learn to drink our cup.

The second way to drink our cup is with the word. It is not enough to claim our sorrow and joy in silence. We also must claim them in a trusted circle of friends. To do so we need to speak about what is in our cup. As long as we live our deepest truth in secret, isolated from a community of love, its burden is too heavy to carry. The fear of being known can make us split off our true inner selves from our public selves and make us despise ourselves even when we are acclaimed and praised by many.

To know ourselves truly and acknowledge fully our own unique journey, we need to be known and acknowledged by others for who we are. We cannot live a spiritual life in secrecy. We cannot find our way to true freedom in isolation. Silence without speaking is as dangerous as solitude without community. They belong together.

Speaking about our cup and what it holds is not easy. It requires a true discipline because, just as we want to run from silence in order to avoid self-confrontation, we want to run from speaking about our inner life in order to avoid confrontation with others.

I am not suggesting that everyone we know or meet should hear about what is in our cup. To the contrary, it would be tactless, unwise, and even dangerous to expose our innermost being to people who cannot offer us safety and trust. That does not create community; it only causes mutual embarrassment and deepens our shame and guilt. But I do suggest that we need loving and caring friends with whom we can speak from the depth of our heart. Such friends can take away the paralysis that secrecy creates. They can offer us a safe and sacred place, where we can express our deepest sorrows and joys, and they can confront us in love, challenging us to a greater spiritual maturity. We might object by saying: "I do not have such trustworthy friends, and I wouldn't know how to find them." But this objection comes from our fear of drinking the cup that Jesus asks us to drink.

When we are fully committed to the spiritual adventure of drinking our cup to the bottom, we will soon discover that people who are on the same journey will offer themselves to us for encouragement and friendship and love. It has been my own most blessed experience that God sends wonderful friends to those who make God their sole concern. This is the mysterious paradox Jesus speaks about when he says that when we leave those who are close to us, for his sake and the sake of the Gospel, we will receive a hundred times more in human support (see Mark 10:29-30).

When we dare to speak from the depth of our heart to the friends God gives us, we will gradually find new freedom within us and new courage to live our own sorrows and joys to the full. When we truly believe that we have nothing to hide from God, we need to have people around us who represent God for us and to whom we can reveal ourselves with complete trust.

Nothing will give us so much strength as being fully known and fully loved by fellow human beings in the Name of God. That gives us the courage to drink our cup to the bottom, knowing it is the cup of our salvation. It will allow us not only to live well but to die well. When we are surrounded by loving friends, death becomes a gateway to the full communion of saints.

The third way to drink our cup is in action.

Action, just as silence and the word, can help us to claim and celebrate our true self. But here again we need discipline, because the world in which we live says: "Do this, do that, go here, go there, meet him, meet her." Busyness has become a sign of importance. Having much to do, many places to go, and countless people to meet gives us status and even fame. However, being busy can lead us away from our true vocation and prevent us from drinking our cup.

It is not easy to distinguish between doing what we are called to do and doing what we want to do. Our many wants can easily distract us from our true action. True action leads us to the fulfillment of our vocation. Whether we work in an office, travel the world, write books or make films, care for the poor, offer leadership, or fulfill unspectacular tasks, the question is not "What do I most want?" but "What is my vocation?" The most prestigious position in society can be an expression of obedience to our call as well as a sign of our refusal to hear that call, and the least prestigious position, too, can be a response to our vocation as well as a way to avoid it.

Drinking our cup involves carefully choosing those actions which lead us closer to complete emptying of it, so that at the end of our lives we can say with Jesus: "It is fulfilled" (John 19:30). That indeed, is the paradox: We fulfill life by emptying it. In Jesus' own words: "Anyone who loses his life for my sake will find it" (Matthew 10:39).

When we are committed to do God's will and not our own we soon discover that much of what we do doesn't need to be done by us. What we are called to do are actions that bring us true joy and peace. Just as leaving friends for the sake of the Gospel will bring us friends, so too will letting go of actions not in accord with our call.

Actions that lead to overwork, exhaustion, and burnout can't praise and glorify God. What God calls us to do we *can* do and do *well*. When we listen in silence to God's voice and speak with our friends in trust we will know what we are called to do and we will do it with a grateful heart.

Silence, speaking, and acting are three disciplines to help us to drink our cup. They are disciplines because we do not practice them spontaneously. In a world that encourages us to avoid the real life issues, these disciplines ask for concentrated effort. But if we keep choosing silence, a circle of trusting friends to speak with, and actions that flow from our call, we are in fact drinking our cup, bit by bit, to the bottom. The sorrows of our lives will no longer paralyze us, nor will our joys make us lose perspective. The disciplines of silence, word, and action focus our eyes on the road we are traveling and help us to move forward, step by step, to our goal. We will encounter great obstacles and splendid views, long, dry deserts and also freshwater lakes surrounded by shadow-rich trees. We will have to fight against those who try to attack and rob us. We also will make wonderful friends. We will often wonder if we will ever make it, but one day we will see coming to us the One who has been waiting for us from all eternity to welcome us home.

Yes, we can drink our cup of life to the bottom, and as we drink it we will realize that the One who has called us "the Beloved," even before we were born, is filling it with everlasting life.

Conclusion

THE ANSWER

I have looked at many cups: golden, silver, bronze, and glass cups, splendidly decorated and very simple cups, elegantly shaped and very plain cups. Whatever their material, form, or value, they all speak about drinking. Drinking, like eating, is one of the most universal of human acts. We drink to stay alive, or we drink ourselves to death. When people say: "He drinks a lot," we think of alcoholism and family trouble. But when they say: "I wish you could come over to have a drink with us," we think about hospitality, celebration, friendship, and intimacy.

It is no surprise that the cup is such a universal symbol. It embodies much that goes on in our lives.

Many cups speak of victory; soccer cups, football cups, and tennis cups are eagerly desired trophies. Pictures of captains holding a victory cup while being carried triumphantly on the shoulders of their teams are imprinted in our memories as reminders of our excitement at winning moments. These cups speak of success, bravery, heroism, fame, popularity, and great power.

Many cups also speak of death. Joseph's silver cup, found in Benjamin's sack, spelled doom. The cups of Isaiah and Jeremiah are the cups of God's wrath and destruction. Socrates' cup was a poisonous one given to him for his execution.

The cup that Jesus speaks about is neither a symbol of victory nor a symbol of death. It is a symbol of life, filled with sorrows and joys that we can hold, lift, and drink as a blessing and a way to salvation. "Can you drink the cup that I am going to drink?" Jesus asks us. It is the question that will have a different meaning every day of our lives. Can we embrace fully the sorrows and joys that come to us day after day? At one moment it might seem so easy to drink the cup, and we give a quick yes to Jesus' question. Shortly afterwards everything might look and feel quite different, and our whole being might cry out, "No, never!" We have to let the yes and the no both speak in us so that we can come to know ever more deeply the enormous challenge of Jesus' question.

John and James had not the faintest idea of what they were saying when they said yes. They hardly understood who Jesus was. They didn't think about him as a leader who would be betrayed, tortured, and killed on a cross. Nor did they dream about their own lives as marked by tiresome travels and harsh persecutions, and consumed by contemplation or martyrdom. Their first easy yes had to be followed by many hard yeses until their cups were completely empty.

And what is the reward of it all? John and James' mother wanted a concrete reward: "Promise that these two sons of mine may sit one at your right hand and the other at your left in your kingdom" (Matthew 20:21). She and they had little doubt about what they wanted. They wanted power, influence, success, and wealth. They were preparing themselves for a significant role when the Roman occupiers would be thrown out and Jesus would be king and have his own cabinet of ministers. They wanted to be his right- and left-hand men in the new political order.

Still, notwithstanding all their misperceptions, they had been deeply touched by this man Jesus. In his presence they had experienced something radically new, something that went beyond anything they had ever imagined. It had to do with inner freedom, love, care, hope, and, most of all, with God. Yes, they wanted power and influence, but beyond that they wanted to stay close to Jesus at all costs. As their journey continued, they gradually discovered what they had said yes to. They heard about being a servant instead of a master, about seeking the last place instead of the first, about giving up their lives instead of controlling other people's lives. Each time they had to make a choice again. Did they want to stay with Jesus or leave? Did they want to follow the way of Jesus or look for someone else who could give them the power they desired?

Later Jesus challenged them directly: "What about you, do you want to go away?" Peter responded: "Lord, to whom shall we go? You have the message of eternal life, and we believe; we have come to know that you are the Holy One of God" (John 6:67-69). He and his friends had started to glimpse the Kingdom Jesus had been talking about. But again there was that question: "Can you drink the cup?" They said yes over and over. And what about the seats in the Kingdom? They might not be the kinds of seats they expected, but could they still be closer to Jesus than the other followers?

Jesus' answer is as radical as his question: ". . . as for seats at my right hand and my left, these are not mine to grant; they belong to those to whom they have been allotted by my Father" (Matthew 20:23). Drinking the cup is not a heroic act with a nice reward! It is not part of a tit-for-tat agreement. Drinking the cup is an act of selfless love, an act of immense trust, an act of surrender to a God who will give what we need when we need it.

Jesus' inviting us to drink the cup without offering the reward we expect is the great challenge of the spiritual life. It breaks through all human calculations and expectations. It defies all our wishes to be sure in advance. It turns our hope for a predictable future upside down and pulls down our self-invented safety devices. It asks for the most radical trust in God, the same trust that made Jesus drink the cup to the bottom.

Drinking the cup that Jesus drank is living a life in and with the spirit of Jesus, which is the spirit of unconditional love. The intimacy between Jesus and Abba, his Father, is an intimacy of complete trust, in which there are no power games, no mutually agreed upon promises, no advance guarantees. It is only love—pure, unrestrained, and unlimited love. Completely open, completely free. That intimacy gave Jesus the strength to drink his cup. That same intimacy Jesus wants to give us so that we can drink ours. That intimacy has a Name, a Divine Name. It is called Holy Spirit. Living a spiritual life is living a life in which the Holy Spirit will guide us and give us the strength and courage to keep saying *yes* to the great question.

ONE CUP,
ONE BODY

On July 21, 1997, it will be forty years since Cardinal Bernard Alfrink ordained me to the priesthood and my uncle Anton gave me his golden chalice.

The next morning I celebrated my first Mass in the sisters' chapel of the seminary. I stood in front of the altar, with my back to the sisters who had been so kind to me during my six years of philosophical and theological studies, and slowly read all the Latin readings and prayers. During the offertory I carefully held the chalice. After the consecration I lifted it high above my head so that the sisters could see it. And during communion, after having taken and given the consecrated bread, I drank from it as the only one allowed to do so at that time.

It was an intimate and mystical experience. The presence of Jesus was more real for me than the presence of any friend could possibly be. Afterwards I knelt for a long time and was overwhelmed by the grace of my priesthood.

During the nearly forty years that have followed, I have celebrated the Eucharist every day with very few exceptions, and I can hardly conceive of my life without that consistent experience of intimate communion with Jesus. Still, many things have changed. Today I sit behind a low table in a circle of handicapped men and women. All of us read and pray in English. When the gifts of bread and wine are brought to the table, the wine is poured into large glass cups, held by me and the Eucharistic ministers. During the Eucharistic prayer the bread and the cups are lifted up so that everyone can see the consecrated gifts and experience that Christ is truly among us. Then the body and blood of Christ are offered as food and drink to everyone. And when we offer the cup to each other, we look each other in the eye and say: "The Blood of Christ."

This daily event has deepened our life together over the years and made us more conscious that what we live every day, our sorrows and joys, is an integral part of the great mystery of Christ's death and resurrection. This simple, nearly hidden celebration in the basement of our small house of prayer makes it possible to live our day not just as a random series of events, meetings, and encounters, but as the day the Lord has made to make his presence known to us.

So much has changed! So much has remained the same! Forty years ago, I couldn't have imagined being a priest in the way I am now. Still, it is the continuous participation in the compassionate priesthood of Jesus that makes these forty years look like one long, beautiful Eucharist, one glorious act of petition, praise, and thanksgiving.

The golden chalice became a glass cup, but what it holds has remained the same. It is the life of Christ and our life, blended together into one life. As we drink the cup, we drink the cup that Jesus drank, but we also drink *our* cup. That is the great mystery of the Eucharist. The cup of Jesus, filled with his life, poured out for us and all people, and our cup, filled with our own blood, have become one cup. Together when we drink that cup as Jesus drank it we are transformed into the one body of the living Christ, always dying and always rising for the salvation of the world.